BREATHLESS

The Role of Compassion in Critical Care

A Medical Memoir

Ronald Kotler, M.D.

Addicus Books
Omaha, Nebraska

An Addicus Nonfiction Book

ISBN: 978-1-950091-55-3

Typography and cover by Jack Kusler

This book is not intended to serve as a substitute for a physician. Nor is it the author's intent to give medical advice contrary to that of an attending physician.

Library of Congress Cataloging-in-Publication Data

Names: Kotler, Ronald, 1956– author.
Title: Breathless : the role of compassion in critical care / Ronald Kotler, M.D.
Description: Omaha, Nebraska : Addicus Books, [2021] |
Identifiers: LCCN 2021036497 | ISBN 9781950091553 (trade paperback) | ISBN 9781950091645 (EPUB) | 9781950091638 (PDF) | 9781950091652 (KDL)
Subjects: LCSH: Kotler, Ronald, 1956—Health. | Critical care medicine. | Critically ill—Care. | Patients—Care—Biography. | Terminal care. | Critically ill—Biography. | BISAC: BIOGRAPHY & AUTOBIOGRAPHY / Medical (incl. Patients) | MEDICAL / Terminal Care
Classification: LCC RC86.7 .K68 2021 | DDC 616.02/8—dc23
LC record available at https://lccn.loc.gov/2021036497

Addicus Books, Inc.
P.O. Box 45327
Omaha, Nebraska 68145
AddicusBooks.com
Printed in the United States of America
10 9 8 7 6 5 4 3 2 1

For my grandchildren
Aviva, Ari, Noémie, Luca, Amiel, Lilia, Misha, Solal
Seek a path that will bring happiness to you and to those
around you. Choose a life filled with agape, a love that
recognizes and seeks to alleviate the suffering of others.

To my children and their partners
Jenny, Marc, Rachel, Michael, Drew, and Elana
To my siblings and their partners
Kenny, Lois, Mark, Sherry, and Andy

To my parents
Milton and Marion

To my friends
Michael Lowenstein
Louis Weiss, Janice Goldwater, Jeff Dworetz
Florence Nygaard

To my colleagues and mentors
Eugene Lugano, MD; Michael Casey, MD; Harold Rutenberg,
MD; Louis Dinon, MD; Stephen Gluckman, MD; John Hansen-
Flaschen, MD; Michael Buckley, MD; David Sherer, MD; David
Henry, MD; Ed Viner, MD; Michael Braffman, MD; Allan
Pack, MBchB, PhD; Gary Dorshimer, MD

And most of all, to the love of my life, Jane, my soul mate.

Contents

Foreword

There exists a storied history of writers who straddle medicine and literature. These physician authors all share an ability to meld compelling stories with their knowledge of science and the healing arts. In his new medical memoir, *Breathless—The Role of Compassion in Critical Care,* Dr. Ronald Kotler adds to that rich tradition.

Dr. Kotler, a pulmonologist, critical care medicine, and sleep specialist, has written a new work based on his vast clinical experience spanning four decades of patient care and interactions. Born in Pittsburgh and earning his undergraduate degree at Emory University in Atlanta, Georgia, Dr. Kotler went on to graduate from the University of Pennsylvania School of Medicine, in whose system he also did his internship, residency, and fellowship. Not content to limit practice to internal medicine and pulmonary medicine, he earned advanced certification in both critical care and sleep medicine, two specialties that enabled him to broaden both his clinical experiences and his love of teaching. Indeed, it is this continuing love of teaching that lends Dr. Kotler's talents to the present work, where he succeeds in communicating his fascination with the science of the human body, fusing it with the pathos and drama of human illness and suffering.

It is fitting that Dr. Kotler studied chemistry as an undergraduate, for it is through that discipline that he is able, with felicity and ease, to explain the most complex chemical reactions that lie beyond the scope of the human eye. Whether it is the explanation of how hemoglobin unloads oxygen to the tissues, how the lungs and heart work in congress to ensure the supply of life-giving oxygen to the blood, or the mechanisms by which modern pharmacology enables mere molecules to pull patients from death's doorstep, his prose skillfully reveals what is often beyond the ken of most readers.

The book is told from his point of view, and that is a good thing. For what better way is there to relate the excitement and drama of lifesaving medical interventions, thorny ethical conundrums, and medico-legal pitfalls? Each clinical vignette deals with the shared experiences of patients and their families and the physicians and other healthcare staff who watch over them, coupled with the applicable science related to the medical themes therein. You do not have to be a scientist or a person with knowledge of medicine to appreciate the wonder and fulfillment inherent in the stories. All you must do is read and pay attention.

With the public's eye now more than ever riveted to medicine, health, and healthcare, I have no doubt that *Breathless* will be a welcome addition to your reading. In fact, with so many "bad" stories in the news today, these inspirational stories will, I believe, succeed in brightening your outlook and augmenting your hope and faith in the resilience and strength residing in those who care for all of us—the doctors, nurses, and other professionals who make up what we call the American healthcare system.

Read and be entertained.

David Sherer M.D.,
Chevy Chase, Maryland

Introduction

My world is a hospital, but not just any hospital. It is Pennsylvania Hospital, the nation's first, founded in 1751 by Benjamin Franklin. The hospital is based upon principles of compassion and tolerance as a refuge for the sick and injured, including the poor and what were then labeled as "the insane."

Every day, I witness the compassion and tolerance, envisioned by Ben Franklin, as nurses, doctors, physical therapists, and other healthcare professionals work tirelessly to help those who are ill or dying. I witness the pain of families as they experience the roller coaster ride of critical illness in modern-day intensive care units. I observe the skills of physicians who provide care, decrease suffering, and help families come to terms with end-of-life issues such as withdrawal of life-sustaining medical devices, advances in medicine unthinkable a century ago.

As a medical student, I began to appreciate the complexities of human life from an intellectual perspective. Courses in physiology and biochemistry opened my eyes to the incredible events occurring at a cellular level. I learned how a complex human could grow and thrive in an environment rich in sunlight, water, and oxygen. In college, I learned that over a period of billions of years an environment initially rich in carbon dioxide produced vegetation that survived by converting energy from sunlight and carbon dioxide into an environment rich in oxygen. With the release of massive amounts of oxygen into the earth's atmosphere, human life could then evolve as we know it today.

The oxygen we often take for granted enters deep into the body with each breath we take. This, in conjunction with glucose, a simple sugar in our diet, allows us to produce energy at a cellular level to maintain body heat at a perfect 98.6 degrees Fahrenheit and fuels cellular functions of highly specialized organs. Although billions of cells in an individual share the same genetic information, only certain segments of chromosomes are activated in specific cells. A cell in the liver, for example, has certain segments of chromosomes activated to become liver cells, capable of producing proteins necessary for daily liver function.

Cells in the heart containing the same genetic information have specific chromosomal segments activated so that proteins can be produced to manifest as heart cells that, when working with other heart cells, are capable of rhythmically pumping blood containing oxygen to all the cells of the body. Through a complex network of blood vessels, the human heart provides life-sustaining oxygen along with a constant supply of glucose so that individual cells produce energy in the form of adenosine triphosphate (ATP), the high-energy substance that is needed to fuel all bodily functions.

As a physician with years of education related to cellular function and the cooperative nature of complex human organs, I have watched as diseases have unraveled these intricate processes. I will always marvel at modern medicine, including infection-fighting antibiotics that fight virulent microorganisms. I am amazed also by clot-busting drugs that restore blood flow to vital organs. I observe highly advanced procedures as surgeons remove damaged segments of diseased organs that would otherwise doom a patient. I have observed the suffering of patients and families as they struggle to overcome the adversity of disease. I have witnessed the remarkable capacity of the human body with its tremendous ability to heal and regenerate.

I hope this book will engage patients, practitioners, and the general reader in a way that will lead to better understanding, communication, and decision making, and, ultimately, better outcomes. I have tried to include both technical terms for

Introduction

practitioners as well as common-sense explanations that will be more familiar to patients and families.

I hope that, in a small way, this book will advance the cause of empathy and greater appreciation of the marvels of the human body. I hope, too, that we all realize that life itself is a miracle and how precious and fragile it is.

In this book, I will share stories of patients who have entrusted me with their care during critical moments of their lives over a span of almost forty years. For privacy reasons, I have gone to great lengths to de-identify patients by changing names, merging characters and adjusting biographies. Although each chapter was inspired by one or more patients I had the great privilege of caring for, specific dialogues were modified to further protect the confidentiality of patients and their loved ones. Where these efforts were less than certain to ensure privacy, relevant portions of the manuscript were reviewed with the patient and loved ones and permission to publish was obtained.

Finally, I also focus on ethical issues and the process by which I and other practitioners make decisions on critical issues. Such issues are an important aspect of modern medicine.

1

Thump

The year was 1982, and I was a lowly medical intern working the night shift in the emergency room. In those days, we did not have seasoned, board-certified, emergency room physicians by our sides. It was a rite of passage—just me and Rose, an experienced emergency room nurse, and whoever came in through the doors after midnight. It was scary. I knew that my medical resident, with one additional year of training, was just a phone call away. I also knew that she was sleeping and to be awakened only if absolutely necessary.

Just then, a middle-aged man walked through the electronic doors to the emergency room complaining that he had passed out an hour earlier. It was my responsibility to figure out what had happened, how to treat him, and decide whether to admit him to the hospital or discharge him to go home. Rose seemed to know everything. She was the one who guided all new interns through the graveyard shift. She understood the delicate balance of suggesting a course of action without disrupting the traditional doctor-nurse relationship. With her diplomatic style supported by years of experience, she gently recommended appropriate tests or treatments to novices like me.

I did not have to say a word. Rose immediately placed our patient on a cardiac monitor. Passing out, also known as syncope, could be due to a temporary malfunction of the heart's intrinsic pacemaker that sends electrical signals to the heart muscle so that it contracts regularly. Without a rhythmically pumping heart muscle, blood supply to the brain is quickly cut off. This results in loss of consciousness or passing out. If the heart does not resume its contractions, you die within minutes.

1

Suddenly, the patient stopped talking and his eyes rolled back. The look of imminent death was upon him. Instinctively, I glanced at the heart monitor and saw a flat line. Seconds earlier, the monitor had shown the perfectly regular rhythm of a beating heart. There I was with four years of medical school education, but minimal clinical experience, terrified that this patient would die if I failed to respond quickly and correctly.

Then I remembered one of my mentors, a cardiologist who taught me as a medical student. He once told me of a patient whom he had encountered with a similar story. He shared with me how he resuscitated the man with a simple thump to his chest. Without hesitation, without turning to the nurse, without awakening my medical resident from deep slumber, I slammed my fist down on the patient's chest. Quickly, I turned my attention to the cardiac monitor. The flat line was replaced immediately by electrical activity in the form of what we call QRS complexes—the signals of a beating heart, the same wave forms you see on a heart monitor during medical TV shows.

His heart rate was a bit slower than normal, but fast enough to trigger a functioning heart muscle once again. As blood flow was quickly restored to his brain, the patient began to talk. He spoke as though nothing had happened, but something big had happened. His life was restored with a thump on his chest. I used a mildly violent act, which would ordinarily be interpreted as aggression, to restore a beating heart, a thinking brain, a feeling soul.

I instructed the nurse to page the cardiologist on call. My job was to keep the patient alive until the cardiologist arrived. I knew that the patient needed an emergency pacemaker. Because his own internal pacemaker was failing, we would have to insert a device into his heart to replace the electrical activity that had lasted long enough from birth through his journey to our emergency room that night. I did not budge from his bedside until the cardiologist arrived. I had a clear sense of the urgent nature of what was transpiring.

Prior to the cardiologist's arrival, my patient's heart stopped several more times. Each time, one quick thump to the chest restored electrical activity and a beating heart.

Thump

Later that evening, the cardiologist placed a pacemaker and the patient was transported to the third floor of our hospital for further care and monitoring in our coronary care unit.

My night shift continued as I examined and treated other patients. No patient that night or, for that matter, any subsequent night of my career, could compare to this man whose heart stopped repeatedly only to be restored with a simple, quick thump to the chest. An "old school" intervention that, decades later with advances in technology, is rarely even discussed as an option, but one that some of my older cardiologist colleagues knew well.

More than thirty years later, I still find myself wondering about that magnificent night. To this day, recounting the event gives me an exhilarated feeling. It also leaves me with many unanswered questions. Was it just a coincidence that I happened to hear a lecture on this arcane subject? That this patient with faulty electrical wiring came to our emergency room during my night shift? Would advances in science make results less dependent on coincidences like these? To this day, I wonder. Although the answers remain elusive, one thing remained certain: that doctor-patient interaction was a formative experience for me as a young doctor and beyond any other human experience I could have imagined.

2

Compassionate Detachment

At the core of the successful doctor-patient relationship, dating back centuries, is the physician's deeply held belief that all human life has equivalent intrinsic value and all are worthy of dignity. The physician's expression of curiosity helps form a lasting connection with patients and their loved ones. This respectful attachment lays the foundation for a trusting relationship, one characterized by empathy and compassion. Medical decision making in the context of this relationship is based upon the patient's personal values, goals, and priorities. However, in the moment of a life-threatening emergency, transient detachment allows the physician to maintain extreme focus without distraction.

When treating a patient in a medical crisis, there is no internal discussion or extensive reflection on what is at stake. There is only a derangement of physiology that must be addressed quickly. For a doctor, this type of compartmentalization is essential. For now, the part of the brain that is able to focus on the physiology and acute derangement must supersede and suppress any emotion that would interfere with the timely intervention that can mean the difference between life and death. Now is the time to turn on that switch and act quickly.

At this moment in time, the patient's interests become parallel with those of the physician. The patient's wish to live becomes the physician's wish for him. His desire to watch his grandchildren grow becomes the physician's desire for him. His goal to reach old age becomes the physician's goal for him. Whether the urgent situation involves a long-standing patient or one who has just entered the hospital, this precious individual, often clinging to life, becomes the physician's sole

4

responsibility as critical decisions are made. In the moment, there is no time for lengthy deliberation.

Seemingly an oxymoron, compassionate detachment is a vital attribute of the highly effective healthcare provider. When fears and anxieties about making a catastrophic mistake begin to surface, it is essential to maintain calm competence without arrogance; not just a façade but a steadiness that penetrates to the core and allows for optimal decision making during moments of clinical crisis. Certainly, the acquisition of wisdom, knowledge, and experience with aging helps to guide the clinician down the winding path of decision making during time-sensitive, life-threatening emergencies. But whatever the level of wisdom and experience, it is essential that it is brought to bear with a steady and singular focus.

How do medical professionals do this? At the core of the brain is a structure known as the thalamus. You could compare this part of the brain to an air traffic controller who determines which sensory inputs reach the frontal lobe for the decision-making process. Imagine yourself in a busy restaurant where multiple loud conversations are taking place. It is humanly impossible to focus on multiple conversations at once. However, through control by your thalamus, you can consciously decide which conversation to focus on while ignoring the others. As you choose, you may switch your attention from one conversation to the next.

To function effectively as a physician, one must be able to multitask and be able to change focus quickly when clinical situations arise and only return to a prior problem when the newly discovered concern has been adequately addressed. Each new issue might be addressed in seconds, minutes, or much longer depending on its complexity. It is not uncommon for a physician to leave one problem and return later to that same problem as new information surfaces or additional thoughts reach the frontal lobe, perhaps from new processing, or prior relevant experiences, or knowledge acquisition. Each new problem requires intense focus and often quick decision making.

For example, a patient who is experiencing labored breathing, chest pain, or low blood pressure may be at risk for cardiopulmonary arrest within minutes if not quickly and properly managed. If an emergency issue such as this arises, it must be addressed immediately, with complete and detached focus. Once the critical moment has passed, an opportunity to review the events that have transpired, with genuine concern and compassion, will follow.

3

Breathe

Another fundamental in the world of a critical care pulmonologist that applies across emergencies is understanding the miraculous process of breathing. Most of us will spend our entire lives without a conscious awareness and understanding of breathing. Yet, it is this very process that allows us to survive on planet Earth. As plant life evolved over billions of years, our atmosphere became enriched with the diatomic molecule known as oxygen, the vital gas discovered by Joseph Priestley in 1774. As the human species evolved, it developed a symbiotic relationship with plant life.

Humans and plants have lived in harmony for over one million years. Plants produce the oxygen that we breathe into our lungs to make energy. Humans produce carbon dioxide that plants utilize to make their energy through photosynthesis. This harmonious balance is the essence of life as humans and plants coexist.

As a fetus grows in utero, the developing lungs are filled with fluid and not involved in this gas-exchange process. Instead, oxygen is delivered to the fetus through the placenta firmly attached to the mother's uterus. As oxygenated blood enters the placenta, it passes through the blood vessel known as the inferior vena cava of the fetus as hemoglobin-containing red blood cells make their way to the right side of the heart. Rather than journeying to the tiny alveoli in the lungs, the blood is shunted to the left side of the heart through openings known as the foramen ovale and the ductus arteriosus. By shunting blood away from the fluid-filled lungs of the fetus directly to the left side of the heart, oxygen that has already been attached to hemoglobin in the red blood cells may be delivered to all fetal cells for energy production.

When the infant is delivered, either vaginally or by C-section, the umbilical cord is clamped, and the baby generates negative intrathoracic pressures by sucking in air. Subsequently, fluid that had filled the tiny air sacs of the fetus is quickly cleared and the foramen ovale and ductus arteriosus close to allow blood to flow to the capillaries surrounding the infant's tiny air sacs for oxygen and carbon dioxide exchange as seen in the mature adult. These first of many breaths have set the stage for life in an oxygen-enriched environment.

We humans have evolved so our brains ensure we exhale enough carbon dioxide and inhale enough oxygen to survive. Carbon dioxide, a by-product of cellular metabolism, is essentially a waste product that must be excreted. If exhalation through the lungs is inadequate, volatile acids build up in the bloodstream and cause dysfunction of major organs. Extreme retention of carbon dioxide inevitably causes death.

How does the body ensure adequate excretion of carbon dioxide? At the core of our brain, an area called the brain stem contains the medulla oblongata. Within this core structure of the brain is a cluster of cells known as the Pre-Bötzinger Complex, which serves as the pacemaker of breathing. If these cells function normally, as carbon dioxide rises in the bloodstream, an increase in nerve impulses is sent through the spinal cord via the phrenic nerves to the two hemidiaphragms, one at the bottom of each lung. This increase in nerve impulse transmission leads to faster and deeper breathing so that increased CO2 exhalation may follow to return this potentially deadly molecule to its normal range. This process is the ultimate example of homeostasis in the human body. The same well-tuned mechanism is seen in all mammals.

The other major function of the lungs is to inhale oxygen. Oxygen makes up 20.9 percent of our atmosphere and we must breathe in a constant supply to live. At the cellular level, energy sources such as glucose require oxygen as we create a molecule known as ATP. This chemical fuels all cellular functions and maintains body heat. Without it, we die. The brain in particular will cease to function within minutes of oxygen deprivation. The body has fine-tuned sensors that have evolved to make sure we breathe in enough oxygen.

During exercise, oxygen demands increase dramatically as our muscles contract and require increased supplies of ATP. Our physiological response is to breathe deeper and faster. In a deconditioned person who rarely exercises, running will quickly lead to an uncomfortable feeling of breathlessness. In a highly conditioned athlete who runs marathons, cardiovascular changes in the heart's blood vessels and cells develop to allow for the delivery of oxygen more efficiently and with significantly less cardiac effort. The highly conditioned athlete is less likely to experience breathlessness until extreme exercise has been performed. Various disease processes of the lungs and heart can interfere with the process of oxygen delivery and carbon dioxide excretion, and if not recognized and treated, may cause considerable breathlessness, or shortness of breath. Progressive deterioration caused by many of these conditions may lead to death.

We take for granted the oxygen we breathe. Two oxygen atoms, each in search of the other to share electrons in their outer atomic shells, create a strong covalent bond to form what we know as O_2. With each breath, oxygen molecules begin their journey without a road map, compass, or GPS, and yet, these essential molecules routinely travel in pathways of blood vessels through all the cells of our bodies.

As oxygen enters the nose and mouth, it passes through the tracheobronchial airways that are shaped like an inverted hollow tree. As with any tree, its branches divide and become narrower and more numerous. At the end of the minuscule branches, oxygen reaches tiny air sacs known as alveoli. These delicate structures have paper-thin walls that allow gas molecules such as oxygen to diffuse into networks of blood vessels known as capillaries. Once within these branching blood vessels, each molecule of oxygen is scooped up by one of 25 trillion red blood cells swimming through these tubular networks of branching highways.

Each individual red blood cell, like a flexible flying saucer, contains over 200 million molecules of hemoglobin, each of which serves as a humble chariot for four molecules of oxygen. Red blood cells have no motor or energy source for transport. They simply swim downstream in the current produced by a pumping heart. Each red blood cell, with its numerous molecules of oxygen carried by hemoglobin, journeys to human cells in need of its passengers.

All human cells require energy to function. The brain requires oxygen to fuel its highly complex neurons, and muscles need oxygen to fuel their well-coordinated contractions. As we walk and talk simultaneously, we rely on a constant flow of red blood cells to deliver oxygen to fuel our cellular activities. Once at the cellular level, the hemoglobin molecule empties its oxygen-containing chariot. Simultaneously, cells metabolize food into glucose molecules that are then broken down and subsequently transfer electrons to oxygen molecules. These processes, known as the citric acid cycle and oxidative phosphorylation, yield water, but more importantly, produce ATP, the body's primary energy molecule. Without an assembly line constantly producing billions of molecules of ATP, we run out of gas and cease to function.

Every effortless breath from birth to death is a wondrous gift for which we should all express daily gratitude. Unfortunately for many, this great blessing is short lived. For those afflicted with various breathing disorders, each inspiration becomes labored and requires considerable respiratory muscle work. Increased work of breathing may be experienced as an uncomfortable sensation variably described as shortness of breath or breathlessness. Often, the sensation is associated with anxiety and sometimes a sense of impending doom that may be quite terrifying.

We as medical professionals often focus on relieving pain but sometimes underestimate the profound discomfort of difficulty with breathing. In its mildest forms, breathlessness may not be obvious even to the keen observer. In its advanced state, disease that causes breathlessness may manifest with obvious signs of distress characterized by rapid rate of breathing and recruitment of neck muscles to supplement the diaphragm's inadequate efforts to suck in air. The sufferer may appear fatigued, diaphoretic (sweating excessively), annoyed, or terrified. If the respiratory disease progresses without a successful intervention, extreme efforts to breathe may then appear but as fatigue worsens, this marathon race will be followed by a decreasing rate of agonal ineffective breathing, altered sensorium, and ultimately complete cessation of respiratory effort. As oxygen supplies remaining in the lungs become rapidly depleted, the heart ceases to function and cardiac arrest ensues. Without timely resuscitation, death follows quickly.

4

Medical Detective

In searching for the cause of breathlessness, the provider becomes a medical detective attempting to uncover the culprit. Usually, the disease process is easily identified and quickly remedied with an appropriate and timely intervention. Whether treatable or not, emotional and physical suffering can be alleviated to a great degree with compassionate support and, if necessary, for a dying patient, potent narcotics and benzodiazepines to relieve discomfort and anxiety and allow death to proceed peacefully and with dignity.

Causes of breathlessness fall into one or more of four categories:

- *Pulmonary (Diseases of the Lungs):* This category includes diseases of airways that begin in the nose and mouth and travel through branching roads like an inverted hollow tree ending in the tiny sacs known as alveoli. The alveoli are surrounded by networks of blood vessels known as capillaries. These conduits of blood cells are supported by tissue known as the interstitium. Abnormalities caused by disease anywhere along the path of airflow may lead to a sensation of breathlessness.

- *Cardiac (Diseases of the Heart):* The heart and lungs are connected anatomically and physiologically. Various structures of the four-chambered heart muscle may become diseased and lead to a backup of fluids into the lungs, resulting in breathlessness. The heart contains four valves that open and shut in a coordinated manner to allow sequential expulsion of blood to all the tissues of the body. Coronary arteries supply blood-enriched oxygen to the muscle cells for ongoing pumping and electrical activity. A thin sac known as the pericardium surrounds the heart.

- *Neurological (Diseases of the Brain, Spinal Cord, Peripheral Nerves, and Muscles):* Effective breathing requires intact neurological functioning as rhythmic electrical impulses generated in the core of the brain travel rapidly down the spinal cord, through the right and left phrenic nerves, to their corresponding hemidiaphragms situated under each lung. Interruption of this highly regulated pathway of electrical activity at any point may result in breathing difficulty.

- *Miscellaneous:* The fourth and final category includes anemia, which is an inadequate number of red blood cells to carry oxygen, and metabolic disturbances such as acidosis (too much acid in the blood). When cellular function is impaired and acid builds up in the body, the lungs must work extra hard to excrete carbon dioxide, a volatile acid. This may be experienced as shortness of breath. Anxiety, also in this category, may be a contributing factor to the sensation of breathlessness.

Through a detailed history obtained from the patient, physical examination performed by the provider, and testing such as chest X-ray, pulmonary function tests, oxygen saturation level measurement, electrocardiogram, and cardiac echo, most causes of breathlessness become readily apparent.

After a diagnosis is established and with the use of evidence-based medicine, treatment is tailored to the individual and reviewed with the patient. Intervention may include medications such as pills or inhalers, supplemental oxygen through nasal prongs, or placement on a ventilator used noninvasively through a face mask, or invasively through a breathing tube placed in the mouth and advanced through the vocal cords to the windpipe, known as the trachea.

Tremendous advances in pulmonary medicine over the last several decades have led to great improvement in treatment of patients suffering from respiratory diseases. Arguably, the greatest achievement in battling respiratory diseases is the invention of the ventilator, a term that became known the world over as a result of the COVID-19 pandemic of 2020. Whether an invasive or noninvasive ventilator is used, a ventilator is a mechanical apparatus that generates pressure so air flows through a breathing tube to inflate the lungs with various mixtures of nitrogen and oxygen. The combination of these gases may be adjusted so the oxygen concentration is 21 percent, the same as the air we breathe, or concentrations as high as 100 percent, depending on the ability of the lungs to transfer oxygen to circulating red blood cells. A ventilator also helps move carbon dioxide out of the lungs.

The lowest oxygen concentration to maintain adequate delivery of oxygen to all the cells of the body is chosen to avoid toxicity. Continuous monitoring of oxygen levels with another marvelous invention, a finger probe known as a pulse oximeter, allows for an increase or decrease of oxygen concentration provided by the ventilator based upon changing lung function. A progressive need to increase oxygen concentration delivery is consistent with disease worsening. The ability to lower oxygen concentration suggests clinical improvement with a greater likelihood of liberation from ventilatory support. Prior to the advent of ventilators, many patients succumbed to the progressive diseases that today are readily curable.

Necessity is the mother of invention. During springtime in the 1950s, nothing brought more terror into a parent's soul than a child's awakening with a fever. For many of these children, paralytic polio was diagnosed by nightfall. Respiratory failure due to neuromuscular weakness from the viral invasion of nerve cells frequently led to death. Without an adequate source of ventilators, hospitals recruited medical students to place a device over the face of each terrified youth and rhythmically pump oxygen into the lungs and passively allow carbon dioxide to be excreted. Without these efforts, coma and ultimately death ensued due to lack of oxygen and extremely high levels of toxic carbon dioxide. Medical students worked eight-hour shifts in rotation for weeks to save these young, terrified souls.

Government, healthcare professionals, and industry worked collaboratively during the polio pandemic by manufacturing greatly needed ventilators. Ultimately, vaccines developed by teams led by Drs. Jonas Salk (at a time when he lived in the Pittsburgh neighborhood I later grew up in) and Albert Sabin eradicated polio in developed nations. It was the polio pandemic that helped prepare future generations for disasters caused by tiny microbes leading to respiratory failure, advances that became even more important in the COVID-19 pandemic.

5

Uncle Billy

Even his friends called him Uncle Billy. Although he never married and had no children, his deceased brother's three daughters saw him as a father figure. When Bill went for a doctor's visit, one of his nieces always accompanied him, took extensive notes, and asked multiple questions. Bill had been a loving, generous uncle since the birth of his nieces. When his older brother died, he helped them financially and spoke to them by telephone regularly.

None of the nieces had a medical background, but they were very knowledgeable regarding the cancer from which their Uncle Bill suffered. Bill had lived with non-Hodgkin's lymphoma for ten years. Initially quite indolent (not progressing rapidly and causing little pain), the disease progression during the past year had become quite worrisome. Despite multiple attempts with various chemotherapeutic regimens, follow-up CT scans showed progression. The month before I met Bill, his oncologist started a new regimen, hopeful of a clinical response but realistic that long-term disease control was unlikely.

It was a beautiful spring afternoon, and I was hoping to leave work on time so I could watch my twin daughters' tennis match. I always prided myself on rarely missing their sporting events. At 4:00 P.M., my beeper alarmed. This was before cell phones revolutionized communication between healthcare providers. I was requested to perform a consultation on Bill in the intermediate critical care unit.

After having tolerated his last round of chemotherapy with only minimal nausea, Billy had become progressively short of

16

breath. Initially, walking up steps led to mild difficulty. Now Billy was short of breath at rest. I was called upon to provide guidance for his caring physicians but most of all for Bill and his nieces.

After reviewing his medical chart and serial CT scans, I met Bill, a thin, gray-haired man who appeared younger than his age of sixty-five. His nieces Patricia, Ann, and Catherine were sitting at the edge of his bed with looks of great concern. The uncle who had once given them piggyback rides was now weak and thin and showing the signs of chronic disease. His breathing was moderately labored, and any movement led to a quick drop in his oxygen saturation level.

I introduced myself as the consulting lung physician. Ordinarily, I would take my time getting to know the patient as an individual. I had learned through the years that the initial visit was crucial in gaining the trust of the patient. Unfortunately, there was little time for chitchat. Bill's breathing was obviously labored, and timely decisions needed to be made. I asked Bill how he was feeling and what had changed. It was important to get a sense of the pace of his illness. Bill spoke slowly and each sentence was punctuated by a deep breath, but he was able to inform me that his breathing had worsened considerably over the past forty-eight hours.

I faced the challenge of determining quickly what was causing his sudden clinical change and intervening, if possible, to prevent further deterioration. We needed to determine if Bill's worsening was due to a reversible, treatable cause or progression of his refractory non-Hodgkin's lymphoma. The distinction between the two was vital as it would shape my recommendations.

When Bill presented to the emergency room earlier in the day, a CT scan of the chest showed no evidence of pulmonary emboli. This type of scan is frequently performed when searching for the cause of respiratory deterioration in patients with malignancy. Although blood clots in the pulmonary arterial tree are life threatening, we often have a sense of relief when we find them in this setting. It gives us a sense of optimism that we have found a treatable, reversible cause of increasing shortness of breath.

This was not the case for Bill. There was no evidence of fluid surrounding his heart on an echocardiogram. Nor was there evidence of a heart attack or congestive heart failure based on blood tests, chest radiograph, and physical examination. When I asked Bill and his nieces what their understanding of his lymphoma was, Catherine, the older niece, quickly and succinctly reviewed ten years of chemotherapy regimens, temporary responses, and the most recent treatment, as Bill nodded in agreement.

In situations such as this, it is essential to ensure that patients and their loved ones have a clear understanding of the medical facts prior to further discussion. We in the medical profession often do a poor job of educating patients about their illnesses. Inadequate communication between doctor and patient leads to patient mistrust and sometimes unnecessary aggressive care at a time when a focus on comfort care may be in the patient's best interest. I was glad that Bill's family was knowledgeable, articulate, and caring, and that Bill was able to follow along and indicate his understanding.

I explained to Bill and his nieces that there was uncertainty about what was causing his recent decline. I explained that most likely we were dealing with:

- A diffuse lung infection related to his immunocompromised state
- A side effect from chemotherapy known as drug-induced pulmonary toxicity
- Progressive refractory no longer treatable non-Hodgkin's lymphoma

After feeling reassured that Bill had a clear understanding of the trajectory of his non-Hodgkin's lymphoma, I asked him what his goals and priorities were. He recounted that he had lived a great life and was grateful for the added years from chemotherapy but was ready to switch to comfort care unless there was a reversible process with a reasonable chance of treatment response leading to an acceptable quality of life.

For potential infection, broad-spectrum antibiotics had been initiated immediately in the emergency department. For the chance of drug-induced pulmonary toxicity, high-dose intravenous steroids were being given. This left us with the distinct possibility that Bill was dying from progressive refractory non-Hodgkin's lymphoma that had spread throughout his lungs. Patricia, Ann, and Catherine began to sob. Catherine slowly turned to me and in a quiet voice queried, "What would you do if this were your loved one?"

Before answering, I paused and looked at Bill. I quickly assessed his respiratory status. His respiratory rate had climbed to thirty breaths per minute (the normal rate is around twenty). His thinned, deconditioned diaphragm was on the final lap of a marathon. Without rest in the very near future, his diaphragm would progressively fatigue, and he would develop a respiratory arrest.

A quick decision had to be made. Should I suggest comfort care only with Do Not Resuscitate/Do Not Intubate orders following initiation of morphine to allow Bill to die peacefully, attended by his caring nieces? Should I suggest placement of a breathing tube for connection to a mechanical ventilator with the knowledge that Bill might never be strong enough for liberation from ventilatory support? Was it in Bill's best interest to undertake aggressive measures that could sustain his vital organs for weeks and possibly months without a realistic hope of ever resuming a life with quality as he knew it?

This close-knit family had turned to me for guidance and compassion in their moment of greatest need. These four souls were strangers to me. Now they were trusting me to plot a course consistent with Bill's goals, priorities, and disease trajectory in the context of a realistic chance of meaningful recovery.

Medical schools are well equipped to teach human physiology and its derangements leading to disease. Modern medicine has brought us great advances such as vaccines, antibiotics, and gene therapy to name a few.

Now, in this moment, after all the facts were reviewed, Bill and his nieces looked to me for answers. They watched to see how this gray-haired physician would apply what he had learned in only one hour about the man they had loved for a lifetime. How would I exercise this tremendous power bestowed upon me by society in the form of a license to practice medicine? How would I synthesize all the data and make a wise recommendation in the context of the many unknown variables?

I sat at the edge of Bill's bed, held his hand, and gazed into his eyes for a moment. I made it clear that without placement on a ventilator, Bill would likely soon die as his lungs continued to fail. I told Bill that if he chose a nonaggressive approach, we would ensure that he would experience no suffering by placing him on a morphine drip with adjustments as needed, not to hasten death, but to relieve any discomfort, including breathlessness.

I then reviewed with Bill and his nieces my recommendation to insert a breathing tube within the hour and transfer him to the intensive care unit with a plan for a lung biopsy by my surgical colleague. He would be sedated for the procedure while on the ventilator. Furthermore, I suggested that if the biopsy demonstrated a reversible process such as an infection or drug toxicity, we should continue aggressive care at least for a while to see if he improved. However, I suggested that if the lung biopsy showed only non-Hodgkin's lymphoma, as the disease had become progressively unresponsive to chemotherapy, we should remove ventilatory support and proceed with comfort care only.

After Bill glanced briefly at his three nieces, he responded, "Sounds perfect." His nieces all nodded in agreement. I told Bill and his nieces I would leave the room and allow them some quiet time. In my heart, I knew most likely these would be their final meaningful moments together. Their last chance to hug, say good-bye, express gratitude for having shared so much over so many years.

I went to the nursing station to coordinate care. I reviewed plans with the head nurse, the medical intern, and the referring primary care provider. I called the surgeon to secure a place on the OR schedule for the lung biopsy. I notified the ICU resident to facilitate transfer. Lastly, I called anesthesia and asked them to join me in Bill's room for placement of a breathing tube to initiate mechanical ventilation.

I returned to inform Bill and his nieces that anesthesia would arrive within minutes. This left the family a last chance for hugs and kisses and wishes for good luck. I informed the nieces that we would meet the next afternoon in the ICU waiting room for an update.

I peeked at my watch and was surprised that two and a half hours had passed so quickly, and it was already 6:30 P.M. Surely, I had missed my daughters' match. When I arrived home that night, I was met with open arms. I apologized for missing the tennis match and hugged my wife and children a bit tighter and longer than usual.

Bill's surgical biopsy went quite well. During this procedure, the surgeon made a small incision to obtain a two-inch-by-two-inch piece of lung tissue while using the most recent CT scan of the chest as a road map. It was important for the surgeon to obtain a representative sample of tissue for evaluation. I visited Bill post-op in the intensive care unit.

This man, who lived and loved and was loved in return, lay there peacefully with a breathing tube in his mouth and a surgical tube emanating from the left side of his chest. He was heavily sedated and showed no signs of distress. Compression devices on his calves pumped sequentially to prevent formation of blood clots postoperatively. He was at substantially increased risk for clot formation because of his malignancy, immobilization, and postoperative state. Ironically, patients often die in the ICU not from the primary process that led to respiratory failure but from a nosocomial (hospital-acquired) problem such as pulmonary embolism or life-threatening infection. I reviewed the ventilator settings and ensured that Bill was getting adequate oxygen at a nontoxic concentration.

The ICU waiting room was filled with family and friends of loved ones who were critically ill, either stable or unstable. The intensive care unit often is a roller coaster ride, with peaks of joy as patients improve and troughs of dread as patients decline. Death can come quickly as clinical deterioration may present without warning. Nothing in life prepares a patient and loved ones as they anxiously await any piece of news, any bit of hope that they will be reunited with their loved one in a time of better health.

My meeting that day with Bill's nieces was very brief. I reviewed that the surgery went well, and their uncle was stable. We planned to meet again the following afternoon. By then, I could review results of the lung biopsy. I asked if there were any questions and as there were none, I nodded and left for the office to see my outpatients.

The following afternoon at 1:00 P.M., I met with the pathologist and several of her residents to review Bill's biopsy slides using a multiheaded microscope. As Dr. Davis completed her review, I knew my suspicion was correct. Bill's lungs showed no evidence of infection or drug toxicity. Widespread lymphoma was penetrating his delicate air sacs. His breathlessness was due to the endless procession of roadblocks created by cancer cells multiplying out of control. These masses of deadly tissue were preventing oxygen molecules from diffusing into the clusters of capillaries surrounding his alveoli. There was no reasonable hope of recovery.

I went to the elevator and headed for the third floor. When I reached the ICU waiting room, I saw many unfamiliar faces. Bill's nieces were not there. I knew I could find them at Bill's bedside. When I entered the ICU, I heard the usual blare of alarms sounding and witnessed the intersecting paths of healthcare providers rushing to meet the needs of critically ill patients with various diseases.

I peered through the glass door of Bill's ICU room for a moment. I observed a scene of gentle kindness. Bill was attended by his nieces looking lovingly on this man who had helped raise them. When they saw me, I motioned for them to join me in the ICU conference room. I could not disguise the disappointment in my eyes. They knew they were losing this wonderful man who had brought so much joy into their lives.

As we sat, I explained the results. I told them we would proceed with removal of the breathing tube and focus on comfort care only. They nodded in agreement. The process we had agreed upon while Bill was still able to express his wishes relieved his nieces of the often-unbearable burden of surrogate decision making. The decision had already been made by Bill. Now our responsibility was to proceed with his previously expressed wishes.

At that moment, I recalled that during my fellowship training in 1985, my mentor bestowed upon me the skill of discussing advance directives, end-of-life care, and issues regarding withholding or withdrawing life support. These discussions ideally occur in the office setting in the context of a long-term doctor-patient connection during a time of clinical stability, but unfortunately, such conversations often occur at a time of acute medical crisis between a doctor and a patient with a newly formed relationship.

This suboptimal approach raises many challenges. How can a doctor advise a patient he has never met before? Who never had an adequate opportunity to learn about the patient's life, family, interests, goals, and priorities? How is the patient able to develop trust quickly for a total stranger in a white coat? With the rapid development of the palliative care field, we healthcare providers are getting better at initiating earlier discussions that will better serve our patients and their wishes and decrease futile healthcare delivery often provided in ICUs in the final moments of life.

By inappropriately asking the patient or loved one the open-ended question, "Do you want us to do everything?" we miss an opportunity to guide them with knowledge compassionately applied and focused on the interests of the patient. Listening to patients and grasping their understanding of the disease process, while gently helping them and their families gain prognostic awareness, and then making specific recommendations consistent with their goals and priorities, allows us as healthcare providers to fulfill our greatest responsibility as we walk this tortuous path together.

This approach, although always leaving opportunity for the patient to question and disagree, is almost always well received, and often significantly relieves the burden and anguish for the patient and family. Ultimately, the competent adult, or his or her surrogate, has the privilege/right of decision making. We as providers are best suited to guide with knowledge, experience, and compassion in the context of the patient's goals, priorities, and personal beliefs.

As Bill's nieces had kept vigil all night, each had an opportunity to say good-bye. Catherine asked me how long I thought Bill would survive without a ventilator. I told her it was difficult to know but that in my experience, it could be minutes or even days but not likely longer.

I instructed the respiratory therapist to change the ventilator mode to minimal support. This gave us an opportunity to see if Bill required an increase in intravenous morphine to relieve the discomfort that might follow removal of the breathing tube as his weakened, debilitated lungs assumed all responsibility for breathing. Indeed, within minutes of changing the ventilator mode, Bill became extremely tachypneic (excessively rapid breathing) with a markedly increased respiratory rate, a sign that his debilitated body was no longer able to breathe on its own.

Though his level of sedation with Propofol suggested lack of awareness, we increased his morphine drip until he appeared to be breathing peacefully with minimal ventilatory support. Once we were confident that Bill would not endure any breathlessness, we removed the breathing tube and turned off all monitors. There was no need now to watch Bill's plummeting oxygen level or dropping heart rate. There was no benefit from hearing alarms sounding in response. To the contrary, these monitor alerts that normally summon help would now only contribute to distress for his nieces. He was dying. He was at peace. His death could come with dignity and comfort, and he was surrounded by loved ones. I went to Bill's ICU room for a last discussion with Bill's nieces. I told them that they should stay by his side, hold his hand, and share memories. Bill died peacefully several hours later.

Successful liberation from mechanical ventilation following sufficient favorable resolution of an acute illness is a joyous moment for the patient, family, and the medical team. However, in the context of end-of-life compassionate removal of ventilatory support, as was the case with Bill, death is often hastened. Medical societies, ethicists, and legal scholars generally concur that no distinction should be made between withholding and withdrawing life support because they are considered indistinguishable from a moral perspective. However, to the loving family who has held vigil at the bedside, and to the dedicated healthcare team who have bonded with the patient as they worked tirelessly in an effort to save a human life, there is a strong emotional component. The experience of removing a patient from life support may be profoundly different from that of withholding life support and may lead to significant psychological effects for family and healthcare providers as well.

Uncle Billy

Although a physician is under no obligation to provide a treatment or intervention that she or he deems to be futile, informed consent regarding withholding and withdrawing life support should, nonetheless, be obtained. The patient's perception of futility and the dynamic balance between benefit and burden of a treatment or intervention may not be the same as the physician's due to a difference in personal beliefs and values shaped by life experiences, faith, and religion.

Fortunately, Uncle Billy was able to provide informed consent that allowed initiation of mechanical ventilation when there was potential benefit and subsequent withdrawal of mechanical ventilation when additional information clearly altered the burden/benefit ratio of ongoing life support. His initiation of mechanical ventilation and subsequent withdrawal of mechanical ventilation were in keeping with his previously expressed goals and priorities, as well as his right to autonomy.

———

In accordance with the expressed wish of a patient or the patient's surrogate, a physician may legally withhold or withdraw life support. Medications, such as potent narcotics and benzodiazepines, may legally be given in an effort to relieve suffering from pain, breathlessness, and anxiety at the end of life as long as the primary intention is to relieve suffering. Although these interventions may hasten death as a secondary effect, in the absence of intent to hasten death, it is legal throughout the United States and considered ethically acceptable. Physician-assisted dying is when a physician provides a lethal dose of a medication that the patient administers at his or her chosen time.

The U.S. Supreme Court has declared that the decision to allow physician-assisted dying should be left to each individual state. Eight jurisdictions, including Washington, D.C. and seven states, have legalized physician-assisted dying. It is illegal throughout the United States for a physician to directly administer drugs or toxins with intent of ending a life, even if it is the expressed wish of a patient or patient's surrogate.

Where we are fortunate to be able to have an agreed-upon process reflecting the wishes, priorities, and values of the patient, the loved ones have a better chance to be at peace. Several years after Uncle Billy's death, one of his nieces approached me when we coincidentally crossed paths on the hospital grounds. She reminded me of the events that had transpired and expressed her gratitude for the path we chose during her beloved uncle's moment of medical crisis.

6

Dangerous Clots

Janice knew her body well. Even though the emergency department physician said it was just a cold, she suspected something more serious. When her hemoptysis (coughing up of blood) persisted, she decided to present to our emergency room for a second opinion. As a pulmonary physician, it is not uncommon to provide consultation on a patient coughing up blood. Any hemoptysis needs to be taken seriously as the initial presentation could represent a sentinel (early warning) event that would later lead to death if not adequately evaluated.

Prior to meeting Janice, I reviewed her medical chart. In those days, before electronic health records, papers were clipped together and placed in a bin next to the emergency room clerk's desk. Review of Janice's emergency room documentation indicated that this twenty-seven-year-old healthy female had an unremarkable past medical history and was on no medications. Furthermore, it noted that she had presented with one to two teaspoons of hemoptysis daily for the past week. Her records also stated that she had recently been in another emergency room with an unremarkable evaluation and that she had no symptoms of fever, cough, or chest pain.

Although I hesitated to criticize the work of other physicians, I wondered whether an adequate evaluation had taken place. Had the emergency room physician overlooked something that we might find or did, indeed, this young healthy patient just have a cold, a self-limiting viral illness worthy of just the tincture of time?

As a consultant, I relied on information recorded by other providers and supplemented with additional questions. Before I asked Janice if, indeed, she was on no medicines, I briefly paused and looked at this young female of childbearing age. I wondered, could she be on "the pill?" The development of oral contraceptive therapy has revolutionized women's reproductive rights but not without risk. For a very small minority of women choosing this mode of birth control, blood clot formation has led to life-threatening events. The risk is heightened if the young female smokes or was born with a congenital thrombophilia, an inherited factor deficiency that promotes excessive clot formation.

When I asked Janice if she was currently, or had she recently taken oral contraceptive therapy, without hesitation, she said, "Yes." She had not considered oral contraceptive therapy as a medication. In her mind, medicine was taken for disease and oral contraceptive therapy was for birth control. With this newly found information, and after completing a brief physical exam, I reviewed with Janice my concern for a potentially life-threatening pulmonary embolism, commonly known as a blood clot that affects the lungs.

In patients who are so predisposed, clots form within the deep venous system of lower extremities, known as deep venous thrombosis. These localized leg clots in and of themselves are not life-threatening. However, as clots enlarge, fragments break off and travel up the inferior vena cava, the major vein in the abdomen and chest, and lodge in the pulmonary artery, a large blood vessel branching from the right ventricle of the heart. If the fragments are large enough to obstruct the pulmonary artery as it directs blood flow to the lungs, they can cause a cardiac arrest.

Janice appeared much too comfortable to be close to death. Perhaps the outside emergency department physician was correct. Perhaps this was just a self-limiting viral illness that did not require additional evaluation. Had it not been for the history of oral contraceptive therapy use, I would have agreed. Did the outside emergency department physician know of the oral contraceptive therapy history? Had this vital piece of information been considered in the differential diagnosis of hemoptysis when she was previously evaluated?

When asked, Janice informed me that her recent evaluation had not included a workup for blood clots. Additionally, Janice indicated that she had not mentioned her history of oral contraceptive therapy use, nor had she been asked. We transported Janice to the radiology department for a ventilation perfusion lung scan. The year was 1989 and, in those days, a diagnosis of pulmonary embolism was confirmed by asking the patient to inhale one radioisotope to assess lung ventilation while another isotope was being injected into a vein to assess pulmonary artery perfusion. This was well before CT scanning for blood clots became the first-line imaging technique.

On the lung scan, if ventilation was preserved but perfusion was blocked, the presence of a clot in the pulmonary artery was presumed. Within minutes, I received a call from the radiologist that Janice's study demonstrated multiple bilateral perfusion defects with preserved ventilation. The diagnosis of multiple pulmonary emboli was established. With only minimal hemoptysis and no shortness of breath or chest pain, Janice was experiencing multiple life-threatening pulmonary emboli. The clots had undoubtedly originated in her legs and journeyed to her pulmonary arterial tree. The issue was not so much the emboli she had already endured but the next one that could break off and kill her.

When Janice returned to the emergency department following her lung scan, she appeared quite different. She was now diaphoretic (sweating heavily) and looked frightened. She and I both knew that something had changed. Since her short trip down the hall for her scan, additional clots had dislodged from her legs and traveled to her pulmonary artery. Perhaps one more clot would prematurely end the life of this young woman.

For a moment, I thought about my young twin daughters and considered the possibility that this could one day happen to them. I wondered whether, if one of my daughters had presented to a physician with mild hemoptysis, the provider would make the vital connection between hormonal therapy used for contraception and blood clot formation? I knew that diagnoses were often about context.

Nonspecific symptoms needed to be viewed in the context of risk factors. As a young female on "the pill" with hemoptysis, pulmonary embolism needed to be considered. This was the type of case where a miscommunication could lead to a disastrous result. I was glad to have asked the question, despite a record showing a negative sign next to medications.

Janice's vital signs upon return to the emergency room were markedly worse and she was now complaining of shortness of breath and chest pain with each inspiration. Her blood pressure had dropped to 70/40, very low even for this young patient. Her hypotension (low blood pressure) was undoubtedly due to recurrent embolization that had occurred as she was transferred to the radiology department for her confirmatory study. Should I have initiated treatment when I first suspected pulmonary embolism? Would it have been appropriate to start a blood thinner in a patient coughing up blood before establishing the diagnosis of blood clots? Having thought of a possible cause that previously may have been missed, would this young woman nevertheless die on my watch?

This was the uncertainty I lived with—the day-to-day decision making guided by evidence-based medicine through the lens of experience in the context of a patient's unique set of circumstances. Decision making requiring the intense focus and compartmentalization discussed earlier. Just as we physicians enjoy the gratitude expressed following a good outcome, so we dread the extreme emotional pain brought about by an unexpected demise. One that perhaps could have been prevented if every snap judgment had been exactly right.

I instructed the emergency room nurse to rapidly infuse a bolus of fluid intravenously in the form of normal saline solution. With Janice's low blood pressure, starting fluid resuscitation was a reflex. However, I knew that excessive fluid could enlarge her right ventricle which would then compress the neighboring left ventricle and diminish left ventricular outflow of blood, thereby worsening Janice's hypotension. If this intervention led to no significant improvement in blood pressure, we would initiate therapy with intravenous Levophed, a potent pressor agent that squeezes blood vessels and enhances the contractility of the right and left ventricles.

Janice's blood pressure continued to drop. Now at 65/40, her heart rate was racing to augment her cardiac output and preserve her oxygen delivery to the vital organs of her body. As Janice developed an ashen, pre-death appearance, she said, "Please don't let me die." The Janice who, an hour earlier, looked to be the picture of health was at risk of dying at any minute.

We infused a lytic agent (clot buster) as I silently said a prayer, "God, please don't let her die." At that moment, as I grasped Janice's sweaty hand, I told her "We will get through this. You will be okay." Was I less than truthful? In fact, I did not know with certainty whether or not she would survive the next hour. I was not sure that she would ever see her loved ones again. I did not even know who her loved ones were.

Here was a stranger entrusting me with her life, trusting me to make all the right decisions without delay. Was I worthy of her trust? At that time, I had been an attending physician for only two years. Despite many years of training, I was still young and learning the skills of my trade. Would she have been better served by a more seasoned, experienced physician at that moment in time? Or did coincidence bring her to this intersection with a stranger who possessed adequate skills and knowledge and experience necessary to save her life? There would be time to reflect, and agonize, over these questions. But that time was not now.

By this time, multiple nurses and doctors had joined me at Janice's bedside. We all knew that cardiopulmonary arrest could soon develop, and we wanted to be prepared should resuscitation become necessary. While continuing to hold Janice's hand and not knowing whether the moisture I felt was her sweat or mine, my eyes were fixated on the cardiac monitor. If the clot buster were to work, surely a change in blood pressure or heart rate would soon become evident. The room was quiet. Perhaps the calm before the storm. Was the tornado of cardiopulmonary arrest and resuscitation efforts to follow about to sweep the room?

And then, after a few moments that felt like an eternity, the monitor revealed improvement in Janice's heart rate: 140 decreased to 130, decreased to 120, decreased to 110. I said a silent thank you to God. I knew that the clot buster was dissolving these aggregations of red blood cells that were blocking blood flow in the vital vessels connected to Janice's heart.

Was I thanking God for saving this young soul or was I expressing gratitude for sparing me the unbearable weight brought about by the unexpected death of a patient, a young patient who otherwise might live on for decades? Truthfully, it was probably some of both. I asked the nurse to check Janice's blood pressure. Amazingly, it had normalized. We immediately turned off the Levophed drip as it was no longer needed for blood pressure support. Janice's intense sense of impending doom had resolved. The sweat dripping from her forehead and the look of panic had been replaced by the calm demeanor she had presented with just hours earlier.

I saw Janice daily during her weeklong hospitalization. As we adjusted her blood thinners, she became more animated and briskly walked the hall of her hospital floor. I encouraged Janice to find an alternative method for birth control and referred her to a hematologist for evaluation of a congenital abnormality that might have predisposed her to clot formation. Additionally, an inherited protein deficiency or mutation could impact family members as well.

Venous thromboembolism is a heterogeneous disease process that, when untreated, has a high risk of death. Clot formation in an affected individual typically begins in the deep venous system of the lower extremities. Predisposing risk factors for clot formation include obesity, surgery, immobilization, malignancy, hormonal therapy, hip fracture, and hypercoagulable states such as congenital thrombophilias including certain protein deficiencies. Although many patients will describe unilateral leg pain or swelling as an initial manifestation of clot formation, quite often there are no leg symptoms but only the symptoms related to clot that travels from a leg vein to the pulmonary artery in the chest.

This event is known as a pulmonary embolism. Symptoms of pulmonary embolism include chest pain, shortness of breath, coughing up blood, or blacking out when the clot is quite large. A CT scan of the chest is often performed to confirm the presence of a clot in the pulmonary artery. Fortunately, most patients when diagnosed early are successfully treated with an anticoagulant for three months if a reversible cause is evident or long term if the clot was unprovoked. In the small subset of patients who develop a massive pulmonary embolism manifesting as shock, a lytic clot buster may be used to rapidly dissolve the clot and restore hemodynamic stability. In patients deemed unsafe for a clot buster because of recent surgery or internal bleeding, an embolectomy (surgical procedure to remove a blood clot) performed by an interventional radiologist or a cardiac surgeon may be lifesaving.

Our last interaction on the day of discharge was brief. Perhaps it was briefer than one might expect based upon the events that we had shared. Circumstances that had brought two strangers briefly down a path of common interests would now lead to divergent paths as we continued with our lives.

I never saw Janice again. More than thirty years later, as I watch my young daughters, who are about the age Janice was when she came to our ER, I hope that Janice has gone on to live a healthy and happy productive life. I hope, too, that her life has been filled with all the joys that I have come to know as a parent and grandparent.

7

Sickle Cell Crisis

Sickle cell anemia is an inherited disease, primarily affecting those of African descent. With onset of symptoms early in childhood, and continuing into adulthood, severe disability may result from chronic pain and multiple organ dysfunction. Profound, acute agony can be triggered by dehydration, cold weather, stress, infection, or exercise. Often, however, the trigger is not identified. The suffering patient enduring an acute painful crisis often seeks medical attention in a doctor's office or in the emergency department.

The cause of this profoundly acute, painful crisis is due to a sudden alteration in the shape of the spherical red blood cells. The cells become shaped like a sickle or crescent. These sickled red blood cells stick together and block blood flow through small blood vessels. Tissues served by these blocked blood vessels are deprived of oxygen.

Painful sickle cell crises beginning in early childhood rendered Evelyn sensitive to the pain and suffering of others. She was determined not to let this painful disease define her.

As she went through college and law school, she faced struggles on many fronts. The financial burden, although significant, was less of a challenge than missed classes during painful crises. With determination and family support, she graduated from law school and turned down lucrative opportunities and instead joined a nonprofit organization aiding those with disabilities. Her husband, an engineer, was very supportive as Evelyn endured many painful crises and hospitalizations.

In one such painful sickle cell crisis, Evelyn lapsed in and out of consciousness while on her IV narcotic drip. During lucid moments, her anger mounted as she questioned whether years of institutional racism contributed to underfunding of research for a cure for her sickle cell anemia. As increasing pain and emotional distress overwhelmed her, she pressed the button on her patient-controlled analgesic pump for a bolus of Dilaudid. As this potent narcotic infused into a vein in her arm, it quickly led to a state of calm. She closed her eyes and drifted back into temporary unconsciousness.

Sickle cell anemia likely evolved in Africa as a protection from deadly malaria and serves as a metaphor for the intense pain and suffering passed down through generations of African-Americans as a remnant of the horrific institution of human bondage and ongoing racism. Four hundred years after enslaved Africans arrived on North American shores, the disparities in access to healthcare and treatment based upon race still persist.

Evelyn's nurse, Tom, assessed her frequently through the night to ensure adequate pain control without causing harm. Inadequate narcotic dosing would lead to suffering from the intense pain caused by sickled cells throughout her body. Excessive dosing could cause respiratory depression and death. At 3:00 A.M., Tom gently examined Evelyn and noted normal respiration, heart rate, and blood pressure; however, when he placed a pulse oximeter on her finger, he was alarmed at the very low reading of 75 percent. Normal is 95 percent or above.

Initially, Tom believed it was an error as Evelyn appeared to be breathing quite comfortably. He assumed that such a low oxygen saturation would be associated with signs of respiratory distress. When Tom checked the reading on multiple fingers, the result was the same: profound hypoxemia. Tom realized that Evelyn's lack of respiratory distress in response to a low oxygen level was due to the depressant effect of Dilaudid on receptors in her breathing center. He immediately called the hospital operator through an emergency number and a rapid response team (also known as an RRT) was called.

Within minutes, a swarm of healthcare providers of the RRT appeared at her bedside. An arterial blood gas obtained by drawing blood from her radial artery confirmed the presence of profound hypoxemia. As Evelyn was awakened from her narcotic-induced stupor and told of the need for transfer to the intensive care unit, a portable X-ray machine arrived in her room. Within minutes, her chest X-ray appeared on the computer screen and demonstrated multiple dense white areas in both lungs. It was evident that Evelyn was experiencing acute chest syndrome, a common cause of death in patients with sickle cell anemia. With a 30 percent mortality rate, it was quite possible that she would not live to see her twenty-fifth birthday the following week.

Upon arrival to the intensive care unit, Evelyn did not appear in respiratory distress but now had a fever of 102 degrees. The development of fever to this degree in a critically ill patient is often due to a life-threatening infection. Patients with sickle cell anemia are prone to infection because of the absence of a functioning spleen. Additionally, fever in a patient with sickle cell anemia may be due to widespread diminished flow of oxygen-containing red blood cells to the cellular level. This is characteristically seen in a patient suffering from an acute sickle crisis. She was placed on high-flow nasal cannula to maintain an oxygen saturation of 92 percent to ensure adequate delivery of oxygen to all her organs.

Although the cause of her acute chest syndrome was unclear, potential contributing factors included blocked vessels in her lungs from sickled cells, embolization of fat from her bone marrow to her pulmonary artery, or diffuse pneumonia related to her immunocompromised state with a nonfunctioning spleen, characteristically seen in virtually all patients with sickle cell anemia. Antibiotics were infused and the Red Cross was notified to perform exchange blood transfusions.

Evelyn's blood contained 95 percent of the abnormal hemoglobin S that is the hallmark of sickle cell anemia, and her condition would likely improve if some of her abnormal blood were removed and replaced with blood containing normal hemoglobin A. The goal was to bring her hemoglobin S level down to less than 30 percent of her total hemoglobin. Within hours, exchange transfusions were initiated in her ICU room. Within twenty-four hours, Evelyn felt much improved. Though radiographic resolution lagged her clinical response, within three days she was sufficiently improved clinically and radiographically for discharge home where she would complete her antibiotic regimen, oral narcotics for pain, and initiate therapy with hydroxyurea in an effort to decrease the recurrence of life-threatening sickle crises.

On the day of discharge, the potential benefits of intermittent outpatient exchange transfusions were discussed with the knowledge that her bone marrow would continue to produce abnormal hemoglobin S. The hemoglobin A contained in the red blood cells she received in the hospital by transfusion shared the ultimate fate of all red blood cells: self-destruction within 120 days. Additionally, the possibility of a cure through gene therapy at the National Institutes of Health was reviewed. For the first time during her hospitalization, Evelyn smiled. The prospect of a cure for this awful disease that had caused her so much pain and suffering was a dream come true.

What causes sickle cell anemia, and what is the potential cure that is on the horizon for Evelyn and many other people who suffer from this awful and debilitating disease?

As our bodies rely upon trillions of normally functioning red blood cells to deliver oxygen, marrow in the core of our bones produces 2 million of these Frisbee-shaped cells per second. Two hundred million molecules of hemoglobin are incorporated into each newly minted red blood cell. Every hemoglobin molecule contains four strands of coiled globin protein, each with an iron element at its core, capable of reversibly binding the molecule of oxygen that it can unload to cells for energy production. In normal functioning hemoglobin, known as hemoglobin A, two of these coiled protein strands are known as alpha chains and two are beta chains.

With elucidation of the human genome, scientists have sequenced 3 billion building blocks or nucleotides in our twenty-three pairs of chromosomes containing 25,000 genes that code for all the proteins in our bodies. These proteins determine who we are as individuals.

Genes on chromosome number 11 and number 16 code for the proteins that form the beta and alpha chains of hemoglobin, respectively. Human cells contain twenty-three pairs of chromosomes with half of every pair from each parent.

Chromosome number 11 contains a segment, known as a gene, coding for a densely coiled string of 146 amino acids that form each beta chain of hemoglobin.

In sickle cell anemia, there is a single inherited mutation leading to a change in just one of these amino acids to the amino acid valine rather than the amino acid glutamine. This single alteration in the beta chain amino acid sequence of the hemoglobin molecule alters the configuration of red blood cells as they pass into small veins with lowered oxygen levels during the routine journey back to the lungs.

This destabilization of red blood cells leads to the sickle shape of these floating red Frisbees. The altered shape causes these red blood cells to stick together and obstruct blood vessels, resulting in profound pain and organ dysfunction known as a vaso-occlusive (vessel blockage) crisis. Rather than incorporating hemoglobin A into the red blood cells, patients with sickle cell anemia have red blood cells with the abnormal variant known as hemoglobin S.

When a parent carries the sickle cell gene on one chromosome 11 and the normal gene on the other chromosome 11, he or she is a carrier of the sickle trait but typically unaffected by disease. If a carrier mates with another carrier, sickle cell anemia will develop in any child who inherits chromosome 11 with the sickle gene from both parents. Based on autosomal recessive Mendelian genetic theory, sickle cell anemia occurs in approximately one-fourth of offspring of two sickle trait carriers.

Those in Africa with the carrier state of sickle cell trait have a survival advantage as they are less likely to die from malaria than those without the trait. In an individual who is a carrier with one mutated sickle cell gene, approximately 35–45 percent of their hemoglobin produced contains the abnormal hemoglobin S molecules. This is just enough abnormal hemoglobin S to prevent the deadly malaria-causing parasite swimming in the bloodstream from infecting and destroying red blood cells, but not enough of this mutated hemoglobin to cause destructive and painful sickle cell crises characteristically seen in patients with sickle cell anemia.

In an individual with two sickle cell mutated genes (one from each parent), however, up to 95 percent of their hemoglobin produced is hemoglobin S and this manifests as sickle cell anemia with resultant intermittent painful vaso-occlusive (vessel occlusion) crises and progressive organ destruction, ultimately leading to premature death.

Gene therapy, approved in the United States in 2017, provides hope for the development of treatment that potentially will cure patients suffering from sickle cell anemia. Gene therapy works as follows: After extraction of stem cells from the bone marrow of an affected individual, a modified harmless virus with the corrected gene able to produce normal hemoglobin is presented to the extracted stem cells. Then the stem cells are reinfused into the vein of the patient suffering from sickle cell anemia. If successful, the patient who has suffered so much for so long will now produce normal hemoglobin incapable of causing dreadful, painful crises. This transformative event may one day eradicate sickle cell anemia, surely one of the most painful disease processes ever known to humans, and dramatically improve the lives of patients such as Evelyn.

8

Mr. Woodward

Jeff Woodward was a retired high school history teacher. Mr. Woodward and his wife, who also had been a teacher, lived quite comfortably on their city pensions and Social Security. They both enjoyed volunteering for their local church and teaching English as a second language to local immigrants. City living had kept Jeff and his wife in good physical shape as they walked several miles every day. They did not find it necessary to own a car.

When Jeff developed shortness of breath with activities, however, his wife urged him to seek medical attention. His primary care physician obtained a chest X-ray that revealed extensive abnormalities in the lungs. A CT scan of the chest was obtained and was highly suspicious for a condition known as idiopathic pulmonary fibrosis. His lungs had become extensively scarred for no apparent reason.

Jeff was seventy-five years old when we first met on a hot summer day. He and his wife expressed embarrassment because of the sweat on their shirts. The walk to my office on that sweltering afternoon took longer than usual because of Jeff's exercise limitation, aggravated by the humidity. Their love for each other was quickly evident as they held hands throughout the initial part of the office visit. As I obtained Jeff's history, the doctor-patient relationship solidified quickly. We talked about our children and grandchildren, and our shared interest in baseball, discussing which players were the best. We talked about Jeff's passions, his hobbies, and his undying devotion to his family.

These initial twenty minutes served as the foundation of a trusting relationship that would endure for the next ten years. Although Jeff remained stable for approximately seven years, his exercise tolerance subsequently declined. Once a high school track star, his ability to walk two blocks had become a challenge. This caused great concern for Jeff and Eleanor as they had hoped to enjoy many more years of retirement as city dwellers.

During that initial exam, Jeff appeared comfortable at rest. Examination of his chest with my stethoscope revealed crackling sounds over the bases of both lungs. These sounds reflected the opening of tiny little scarred air sacs with each inspiration. The crackling was a sign of diseased lungs no longer able to deliver oxygen efficiently to the cells of his body.

I placed a pulse oximeter probe on Jeff's index finger. This small device, shaped like an alligator's mouth, provided vital information about his oxygen level by utilizing the physical principle known as spectrophotometric analysis. This is accomplished by passing specific wavelengths of light through Jeff's fingernail. A receptor underneath the fingertip determines how much of one wavelength of light had been absorbed by the molecules of hemoglobin attached to oxygen contained in his red blood cells.

This revolutionary advance in medicine allowed us to assess Jeff's oxygen level accurately while he was at rest and while he was walking. Use of pulse oximetry in the outpatient arena has become of great value in assessing patients with respiratory complaints, and, in the hospital, as an "early warning system" for potential health crises, during surgery for example. Use of pulse oximeters in critical care units has become universal.

Jeff's oxygen assessment by pulse oximetry on that day revealed that while sitting, 98 percent of his hemoglobin molecules were carrying oxygen. A level of 95 percent or above is considered to be within normal limits. A reading of 90 percent or above is adequate to maintain vital organ function.

The next step in my evaluation of Jeff was to assess his oxygenation during ambulation. After all, Jeff did not complain of shortness of breath at rest. His symptoms were only present during activity. With the pulse oximeter on Jeff's finger, he and

I took a walk in the hallway outside my office. Although we talked about our beloved Philadelphia Phillies, I intermittently glanced at the digital readout on the finger probe.

After a few minutes of walking, Jeff's oxygen level dropped to 85 percent. We returned to the office and sat once again. Very quickly, Jeff's oxygen level returned to a baseline level of 98 percent. As I watched Jeff's neck, chest, and abdomen, it was evident that his effort to breathe remained increased following our brief walk. His ability to speak full sentences without intermittent gasps for air was impaired for several minutes as well.

I reviewed the CT scan of the chest with Jeff and his wife. Earlier in my career, I would have lifted a five-pound film holder and searched for an individual black film. Those days were gone. All images are now easily retrieved on a computer screen. Jeff's CT images showed classic findings of a condition known as idiopathic pulmonary fibrosis. The lung images showed a classic "honeycomb" pattern in both lungs.

I explained to Jeff and Eleanor that idiopathic meant no definite cause of disease. Jeff had never been exposed to drugs or chemicals that could cause this abnormality. He had no systemic illness such as lupus or scleroderma that could result in these findings. I explained that Jeff's shortness of breath with activity and his drop in oxygen saturation with walking reflected his body's impaired ability to deliver the tiny molecules of oxygen through the tiny air sacs known as alveoli.

Scarring, or fibrosis, had encircled the air sacs and was interfering with oxygen diffusion to his blood vessels, especially with activity. During exercise, cardiac output is increased and red blood cells swim past the air sacs more quickly. With scarring between the air sacs and the red blood cell–containing blood vessels, oxygen molecules do not have enough time to reach and attach to hemoglobin molecules. This manifests as dyspnea (labored breathing) on exertion and exercise-induced oxygen desaturation.

Jeff and Eleanor, being retired teachers, had searched the Internet prior to the office visit. They were well acquainted with the nature of his illness and the limited treatment options available at that time. Jeff asked me how long he would live. I explained that we should not draw conclusions from outcomes of a large group of patients with idiopathic pulmonary fibrosis suggesting a median survival of three years.

It was important to maintain a level of optimism. I explained that there was a range and some with idiopathic pulmonary fibrosis could live more than ten years. It was only through follow-up that we could come to appreciate Jeff's rate of disease progression. I explained to Jeff that his individual situation could not be predicted and that I would see him in the office every three months. I made it clear to Jeff that he should call me sooner if he had any questions or any concerns.

Jeff understood that, although lung transplant was the only possible hope of a cure, a nationwide shortage of donor organs made this option an impossibility at his advanced age of seventy-five. When I offered Jeff enrollment in a clinical trial for drugs being tested, he quickly declined. The potential value of antifibrotic medications in slowing the progression of this disease process had not yet been established. Because of Jeff's oxygen decrease during exercise, I prescribed portable oxygen that he would carry with him for all activities.

Portable oxygen is another important medical advance of the second half of the twentieth century. There is no question that the harnessing and concentrating of oxygen from the air we breathe into aluminum cylinders has prolonged the lives and relieved the suffering of many patients who endure chronic lung disease. In those with an impaired ability to deliver oxygen from the lungs through the alveoli and to the red blood cells for transport to all cells of the body, flow of this life-sustaining gaseous molecule via nasal prongs known as a cannula proves to be quite beneficial in relieving breathlessness and increasing comfort and sense of well-being.

The determination of supplemental oxygen need is achieved by placing a pulse oximeter on a patient's finger while sitting at rest and during ambulation. The widely accepted threshold for supplementation, based on the medical literature, is 88 percent oxygen saturation. Normally, 95 percent or more of the hemoglobin molecules are attached to oxygen. When 88 percent or less of these delivery molecules carry oxygen, organ dysfunction, including cognitive impairment, may occur and may shorten life. In a patient meeting the criteria of having an oxygen saturation of 88 percent or less at rest, with exercise, or during sleep, insurance companies will typically cover the cost of an oxygen supplementation device.

Various delivery systems are available and one is chosen to meet the patient's needs and lifestyle. Portable oxygen tanks generally vary in size from nine inches to twenty-five inches and may weigh four–fifteen pounds. Larger tanks last longer. Pulsed oxygen through a demand valve oxygen-conserving device that gives a bolus of gas when inspiration is sensed by the device lasts longer than continuous flow; however, for some, pulsed oxygen does not provide adequate oxygenation.

Gaseous oxygen is extracted from the air and compressed in green aluminum tanks at 2,000–3,000 pounds per square inch pressure. A release valve with various flow rates may be controlled by the patient to deliver enriched oxygen in an effort to maintain an oxygen saturation of approximately 92 percent at rest and with exercise. As the oxygen is consumed from the tank and the pressure drops to approximately 200 pounds per square inch, a needle on the gauge will demonstrate a drop toward an empty sign, alerting the user of the need to obtain a new tank from the supplier.

Alternatively, a tank may be filled with liquid oxygen. At negative 297 degrees Fahrenheit, gaseous O2 is cooled to a liquid form that takes up much less space and, therefore, allows for smaller tanks that are easier for the patient to carry. For patients with advanced disease requiring more than three liters per minute of nasal oxygen to maintain an oxygen saturation of 92 percent, liquid oxygen is an appropriate choice. When liquid oxygen converts back to its gaseous form, it expands 860 times. If the patient chooses liquid oxygen, a large reservoir container for storage is kept in the home for refills of the portable tank.

A more popular mode of oxygen delivery for the patient with chronic lung disease is a portable oxygen concentrator. These small devices, weighing less than three pounds, are powered by an electric outlet or a battery, and will suck in room air containing 21 percent oxygen and 79 percent nitrogen, compress the gas and pass it through filters that remove the nitrogen, and concentrate oxygen to 95 percent. These devices are equipped with plastic tubing attached to nasal prongs and a purse-like bag for easy portability. The rechargeable battery may provide five hours of oxygen supply.

Travel by air for patients with lung disease may be dangerous. For some, a lung collapse may develop due to changes in barometric pressure. For others, the risk is related to inevitable drops in oxygen levels as the plane ascends to 35,000 feet. At this level, airplane cabins are pressurized to approximately 8–10,000 feet of altitude based upon FAA flight regulations. However, this elevation, despite the pressurized cabin, is high enough to cause life-threatening drops of oxygen levels in susceptible individuals with lung or cardiac disease.

Those who require oxygen at sea level will likely require a higher flow in air flight. Those who do not qualify for oxygen at sea level, based upon the 88 percent threshold, may require oxygen supplementation during air flight if the baseline oxygen saturation at sea level is 89–94 percent. This level is below normal but not typically low enough to qualify for supplemental oxygen at sea level. High-altitude simulation tests may be performed in a hospital setting to determine optimal oxygen flow during air flight by having the patient breathe a reduced fraction of oxygen at approximately 15 percent to simulate the percentage of oxygen one ordinarily breathes during air flight.

According to the Air Carrier Access Act, patients who require oxygen may fly with their own battery-powered FAA-approved portable oxygen concentrator. Typically, a standard form provided by the airline is signed in advance by the ordering physician who determines optimum oxygen flow rates and safety to travel. A written oxygen prescription is also provided to the patient to present to airline personnel at the time of travel. Informed consent also comes into play. The patient is informed of the potential harm of air travel despite the use of supplemental oxygen. The patient is offered the alternative of train, bus, or car travel and ultimately makes an informed decision based upon a review of the potential harm and benefits of air travel.

For those without lung disease, the drop in oxygen level from the normal baseline during air travel typically is not enough to cause harm. If, however, cabin pressure is lost due to a faulty pressurization system or a structural defect such as a hole in a window at 35,000 feet, airplane generators will deliver oxygen through masks that will drop from the cabin ceiling that will last long enough for the plane to descend to a safer level.

As the years passed, I saw Jeff and Eleanor every three months. Each visit started with pictures of grandchildren. Gradually, Jeff's condition worsened. His exercise tolerance declined and his oxygen supplementation requirement through nasal cannula increased. Seven years after diagnosis, Jeff required oxygen twenty-four hours per day. He could no longer walk from his Center City apartment to my office. Cabs and buses became his source of transportation.

On a cold winter day in February, Eleanor called me in a panic. Jeff was laboring to breathe and had developed a fever of 102 degrees. He was coughing up thick green sputum. I instructed Eleanor to call 911 and we met in the emergency room. It was clear that Jeff had developed bacterial pneumonia despite being up to date on all vaccines. Jeff had received the Pneumovax during the year we first met. This vaccine, developed by Dr. Robert Austrian, offered protection against one of the most common causes of community-acquired pneumonia, known as pneumococcus.

Unfortunately, Jeff's pneumonia was due to a bacterium that did not respond to the vaccine. When I arrived in the emergency room, Jeff had already been placed on a mask to deliver 100 percent oxygen concentration. Despite this, his oxygen level by pulse oximetry was only 83 percent. His respiratory rate, normally twenty breaths per minute or less, was markedly elevated at thirty-five. His neck muscles showed frequent rhythmic retractions, a reflection of the struggle to suck in air to breathe, as perspiration dripped from his forehead.

Jeff asked me if he was dying. I told him that, although idiopathic pulmonary fibrosis was an incurable underlying lung disease, his pneumonia was reversible. I asked Jeff what his priorities were and what he feared. With every few words being followed by a deep gasping breath, Jeff responded that he wanted to see his granddaughter finish college in six months. She had chosen to be an educator just like her grandparents. His greatest fear was not being alive to see that glorious day.

After a brief discussion, we agreed that placing a tube in Jeff's windpipe would be best to support his breathing with a ventilator until his pneumonia resolved. We knew that liberation from mechanical ventilation would be more of a challenge because of his underlying idiopathic pulmonary fibrosis.

Jeff was treated in the intensive care unit for one week with ventilatory support. A feeding tube was placed in his nose for liquid nutrition. Antibiotics were infused through an intravenous catheter in his arm. Injections of heparin were administered into the subcutaneous tissue of his belly to prevent blood clots from forming in his legs. This type of clot, known as deep venous thrombosis, commonly forms in critically ill immobilized patients. If not prevented, the clots grow, break off, and travel up through the inferior vena cava to the heart and block its pumping action. Ironically, many patients admitted to the intensive care unit die not from the primary illness leading to the need for critical care but from other disease processes such as blood clots, gastric ulcer bleeding, or blood infections.

Our goal was to treat Jeff's pneumonia and liberate him from mechanical ventilation before he succumbed to a nosocomial, or hospital-acquired, illness. After seven days on the ventilator, Jeff was showing signs of great improvement. Eleanor, by his side at all times, undoubtedly contributed to his clinical response. Jeff was well enough for a spontaneous breathing trial.

For thirty minutes, and under close observation, Jeff's ventilatory settings were adjusted so his breathing muscles did most of the work. We watched his respiratory rate, his oxygen saturation level, and his heart monitor as well as his work of breathing. At the end of the breathing trial, a blood sample obtained from an indwelling arterial catheter in the radial artery in his wrist confirmed that his blood pH, CO_2, and oxygen levels were all within an acceptable range. The breathing tube was removed.

Because of Jeff's underlying lung disease, we knew he was at risk for failing. We knew to watch him closely for signs of respiratory deterioration, signs that would suggest the need to place him back on the ventilator. To decrease the chance of failure, we placed a mask on his face for a non-invasive form of ventilation. Each time he took a breath, the machine would deliver pressurized air to diminish his work of breathing.

Everyone was delighted with Jeff's progress. By day ten, he was able to be transferred to our intermediate critical care unit. He no longer required the one-on-one nursing monitoring capability of the intensive care unit. He had been weaned off noninvasive ventilation as well.

As is commonly the case, especially in elderly, critically ill patients, Jeff became deconditioned. His body's fight against the life-threatening pneumonia had left him extremely weak. A physical therapist began working with Jeff in an effort to strengthen his muscles. A speech therapist helped Jeff to decrease the possibility that his weakened swallowing muscles would lead to choking while eating.

On day twenty-one, Jeff was discharged to a rehab center for further strengthening and recovery. All along this pathway from admission through discharge, Jeff and Eleanor were treated by compassionate healthcare providers who shared their primary interest and their primary goal of recovery from illness. Jeff returned to my office three months later without Eleanor. He ambulated with a walker and carried a purse containing his portable oxygen device. This vibrant man I had met years earlier was now showing the physical signs of advanced disease. His muscles had atrophied, his cheekbones were prominent, and a look of despair had replaced his previously healthy and confident visage.

Jeff had never before come to the office alone. With great sadness in his eyes, he recounted how Eleanor had died suddenly of a heart attack. Jeff and Eleanor had been married for fifty years. They were a unit. They were inseparable soul mates, always holding hands. Although Jeff still derived great joy from his children and grandchildren, the loss of his life partner was more than he could bear. He cried not for his loss of mobility but for the loss of his life partner.

Jeff was now residing in assisted living. Although he felt much better than the day he was admitted with pneumonia, he never returned to his baseline preadmission level, either physically or emotionally. I recalled his top priority of watching his granddaughter graduate from college. I discussed with Jeff that a return to the ICU for mechanical ventilation was probably not a good idea should the need arise. Jeff clearly wanted to avoid another stay in the intensive care unit. He was appreciative of the additional time his ICU stay had given him but the loss of his wife and progressive clinical deterioration made it clear to him and to me that a focus on comfort measures was most appropriate at this time.

As Jeff's disease had clearly progressed, he knew his time on this earth was increasingly becoming very limited. Having been greatly assisted by my compassionate and learned palliative care colleagues, I responded to Jeff's question regarding longevity, "I hope you will live a long time but I worry you will live just months and I hope I am wrong."

How many times have physicians unfairly evaded this important question and misled patients in their moment of great need by responding, "God only knows." In fact, we physicians, based upon experience and evidence-based medicine, quite often are able to provide a more useful answer, one that will allow the patient to share in our understanding of the nature of a terminal illness and its prognosis in general while never removing hope that the individual may be an outlier who will live longer than expected.

I helped Jeff develop what my palliative care colleagues refer to as "prognostic awareness" so that with disease progression, Jeff could contribute in a meaningful way by expressing his wishes as his illness continued to progress. Jeff asked me if he would suffer as death approached. He now feared the sensation of drowning that he had experienced when he developed pneumonia. I assured Jeff that he would not suffer. We talked about the eventual need for hospice as well as the need ultimately for potent narcotics such as morphine and Dilaudid. Benzodiazepines such as Valium and Ativan would also be used if necessary to relieve any anxiety.

When I mentioned narcotics, Jeff insisted that he had no pain. I explained that narcotics effectively treat the sensation of breathlessness as well as pain. Jeff left that day feeling quite comfortable with the plan we agreed upon. I documented in his chart a DNR, DNI status (Do Not Resuscitate, Do Not Intubate) with a plan to involve hospice when Jeff felt the need. I reviewed with Jeff that only he would know, based on how he felt.

Many in the community have the misconception that hospice care is only for the dying cancer patient. In fact, these compassionate, dedicated healthcare providers relieve the physical and emotional suffering of many patients in their final days of life, often in the home setting, surrounded by loved ones. Since the time I took care of Jeff, a great new field of medicine has evolved. The field of palliative care offers emotional and physical support to the chronically ill patient long before their dying days. Evidence in the medical literature now shows that early involvement of palliative care decreases depression, diminishes the likelihood of futile care in an intensive care unit, and may in fact prolong life. I say with great joy that my son has become a palliative care physician.

In the twentieth century, after the polio epidemic of the 1950s, the medical profession became skilled at prolonging life by artificial means in intensive care units throughout the world. However, the wisdom and appropriateness of doing so must be carefully considered. For the dying patient without a reasonable hope of response to aggressive interventions, the more humane approach includes home-based hospice care, surrounded by loved ones.

The trauma of witnessing a death in the intensive care unit may lead to post-traumatic stress disorder (PTSD) in family members. With PTSD, nightmares and sudden unpleasant flashbacks may persist and contribute to great sadness and anxiety for months after the death of a loved one. It can be devastating for a family member to watch as an agitated, dying family member requires wrist restraints to prevent self-harm from trying to remove tubes from multiple orifices. It is the physician's responsibility to guide patients and their families toward or away from use of aggressive interventions based upon patient goals, wishes, and beliefs in the context of realistic outcomes. As disease progresses, prognostic awareness shared with patients and families assists in the often-challenging decision-making process.

It was a Friday late afternoon when my secretary paged me. Jeff was on the phone and his voice was clearly weakened as he spoke softly with sentences punctuated by audible deep breaths. He asked if we could contact hospice. A team of highly dedicated nurses arrived at Jeff's assisted living home. Their goals and interests were perfectly aligned with Jeff's and mine. There was no other goal but to relieve suffering, preserve dignity, and allow death to follow quietly and peacefully, consistent with Jeff's previously expressed wishes. Morphine liquid eased Jeff's perception of shortness of breath. Ativan pills eradicated all anxiety.

I spoke to Jeff the following Monday. His voice was different. The anxious tone had resolved. He spoke more slowly. He paused after each sentence to take a deep breath but there was no sense of distress. When I asked Jeff how he was feeling, he briefly paused and told me of his wonderful weekend surrounded by his eight adoring grandchildren, three loving children, and their incredibly dedicated spouses. His granddaughter's graduation was two weeks away. Jeff told me of his plan to attend.

June 5th was a beautiful spring day. There was no humidity and the temperature was a comfortable 68 degrees. That morning, Jeff looked in the mirror and saw a skinny, pale man, slightly cyanotic (with bluish skin) and wearing nasal cannula oxygen. He thought to himself, I made it! He had taught thousands of students in high school, had a soul mate for fifty years, had raised three wonderful children, and had witnessed the birth of each of his eight grandchildren. He never missed birthday parties of any of his children or grandchildren and today he would witness his oldest grandchild receive her teaching degree from college.

Jeff was transported by van to the ceremony and luncheon that followed. His grandchildren took turns guiding his wheelchair and sitting on his lap. His eyes never lost that joyful look of fulfillment. The look of a man who truly had lived life to the fullest. A man who understood that nothing in life was more important than love. This was a man who knew the limited value of material possessions as well as the infinite value of knowledge applied with wisdom.

As Jeff returned home that night, he knew that his last day on earth was soon to arrive. He had come to accept death and knew that he would lie next to his soul mate for all eternity. Jeff had reached his goal and had come to terms with life's finite nature. He died peacefully three days later surrounded by loved ones who reminisced about how Jeff had made them laugh and now they cried. Most of all, each recalled how Jeff made them feel loved.

Jeff's funeral service revealed the great wealth he left behind. Not a mass of dollars nor a large portfolio of stocks and bonds, but a different type of currency: one of loving relationships filled with caring and compassion. He was buried in the churchyard next to his wife. His tombstone was marked with the word: Agape. This word is a Christian reference to the highest form of love—giving love and kindness without expectation of personal gain, reward, or recognition. This one word described Jeff's primary philosophy of life.

9

The Greatest Virtue: Compassion

It was a time of great optimism. The year was 1945 and soldiers were returning home from Europe and the Pacific. The world had been saved from tyranny. Tom was a kind and sensitive nine-year-old. With a small American flag in each hand, he rhythmically waved to troops as the local parade passed by. Perhaps it was at this precise moment that he developed his deep sense of patriotism. He was very aware that the fathers of many of his friends would not return home. This young gentle soul knew the joy of an intact family, a joy that contributed to his lifelong devotion to generations before him and those that would follow.

Life after World War II was simple for Tom. He had everything he needed for happiness: a loving family, a comfortable home, and plenty of food. He enjoyed working side by side with his father learning to repair shoes and clean hats. By age twelve, he started to take notice of girls. Little did he know that at age sixteen, he would meet Ellen, the love of his life, his future soul mate and partner.

The trolley stop in front of his father's shoe repair store was a place to gather and reflect on the day's work while waiting for the nightly ride home. It was also one block away from where Ellen worked at Woolworth's five and dime department store. It did not take long for Tom and Ellen to form a strong connection. Four years later, they were married in the Catholic Church.

Tom became a volunteer firefighter and worked his way up the ranks to become captain. This brave man received multiple citations for heroic deeds. In 1975, while a refinery burned for eight days, he put his life on the line while eight of his colleagues perished. Years later, he entered a burning building and single-handedly rescued a 275-pound man who lay unconscious, overcome by smoke inhalation. This was the essence of Tom, a man who would sacrifice his life to save another and go to the ends of the earth for his family.

Ellen was the seventh child of a woman she would never know. Her mother died at age twenty-seven, just two days after she gave birth to Ellen. She was raised by a kind uncle and aunt and became a receptionist in a doctor's office soon after marriage. Together Tom and Ellen brought six children into the world.

The intensive care unit experience can be a frightening one for the patient, visitor, or healthcare provider. My earliest memory of working in the intensive care unit was during my medical internship just following medical school. In those days, the specialty of critical care medicine was in its infancy. Although critically ill patients were centralized in a large room with curtains separating the beds, the interns responsible for caring for these patients were often scattered about the hospital. Highly trained nurses caring for critically ill patients would page the intern if problems arose. The problem could be as simple as an elevated blood sugar requiring an injection of insulin or as complex as a patient with acute respiratory failure on the brink of death without a timely intervention.

Ten years after my medical internship, I met Philip, Tom and Ellen's son, in the intensive care unit. By then, I had completed medical residency, pulmonary fellowship, and had five years' experience as a pulmonary/critical care medicine specialist. My meeting with Philip, although purely coincidental, was transformative for me.

Philip loved cars. Following high school, he worked in the auto parts department at a local car dealer. On the side, he enjoyed repairing cars. He depended on his hands to work under the hood. Philip was Tom and Ellen's fourth child; he was twenty-nine when family members noticed that he was dragging his feet and dropping his tools. He tended to minimize health issues and it was not until he began stumbling that Tom and Ellen convinced him to seek help.

The Greatest Virtue: Compassion

A nurse in the family arranged for Philip to see a local neurosurgeon. An MRI revealed a tumor compressing the spinal cord in his neck. The spinal cord is the core of the electrical wiring of the human body. It sends messages from the brain to our arms and legs to synchronize and coordinate movements. The concert pianist relies on. signals to the fingers to allow Beethoven's greatest works to be heard. The Olympic athlete relies on signals to the legs to sprint 100 meters.

As Philip's weakness progressed, the simplest tasks would no longer be possible. The continued growth of this malignancy would eventually cut off not only signals to the muscles in his arms and legs but would also impinge on higher structures such as the brain stem and cause death.

Philip was referred to a prominent neurosurgeon at our institution. Dr. Jamison was a brilliant, modest, and unassuming surgeon who was famous worldwide for his surgical skills. There was never an air of arrogance or condescension about him. He treated all patients with respect and dignity.

Philip's only chance of survival was surgical removal of his spinal tumor. He also knew that surgery in such a delicate area could lead to quadriplegia. Because his tumor was high in the cervical spine, it could leave him unable to move his arms and legs and unable to breathe on his own.

It was a weekday afternoon on the consult service when I received a call from our office that the neurosurgical team had requested help in the postoperative care of Philip. It was my turn in the pulmonary/critical care medicine group to perform the consult after Philip's surgery that day. This is how I met Philip. I had no way of knowing it would be the beginning of a more than twenty-five-year relationship with Philip, his parents, and his siblings.

Philip was wheeled into the intensive care unit late in the afternoon. It had been a long, delicate surgical procedure performed under the microscope by Dr. Jamison. When I arrived at Philip's bedside, he was still sleepy from the effects of general anesthesia. His parents were by his side.

As I began to talk with Philip's parents, it became clear that this was a very close-knit family who would go to the ends of the earth for each other. Without delay, Tom and Ellen asked three relevant questions: Was Philip cured of cancer?

Would he be able to use his hands and feet? Would he need a ventilator to breathe? Clearly, they had awareness of the worst-case scenario, but nothing could prepare them for the twenty-five-plus years to follow.

As it was late in the afternoon and Philip was still very sleepy, none of these questions could be answered on the day we met. We agreed to reconvene daily. I went home that night and could not stop thinking about Philip. My wife and I reaffirmed how blessed we were to have three healthy children. One of the challenges in taking care of critically ill patients is separating work from home life. Being on call meant maintaining a level of vigilance to respond either by phone or in person to immediately life-threatening conditions at any hour. Even when not on call, it was not always possible to leave work behind. I did get better at this separation as I aged.

When I returned to see Philip the next day, his parents were at his bedside. We quickly developed a close, trusting relationship.

Although usually trying to maintain boundaries with patients and families for self-preservation, I allowed Philip's parents greater access than I had allowed most. Although I am very responsive to all patients, Philip's circumstance affected me greatly and I gave his family almost unlimited access, even on my days off. It became understood within our medical practice that I could be interrupted at any time to take a call, even when not on call, for significant concerns by the family. It was this early bond that led to a strong relationship with Philip and his family. It was this common link that led to yearly summer dinners with our combined families gathering poolside at their suburban home.

It quickly became evident that Philip had been rendered quadriplegic. Although he was cured of his tumor, he would never have use of his arms and legs again. The primary issue was whether he would ever breathe again without ventilatory support. The pacemaker for breathing lies deep within the brain in the brain stem. This part of the brain stem automatically sends an electrical impulse approximately every three to five seconds down the spinal cord to the two hemidiaphragms (the muscles that separate the chest cavity from the abdomen and that serve as the main muscles of respiration).

Each time the hemidiaphragms receive this message, they contract and descend into the abdomen in a coordinated manner. This leads to negative intrathoracic pressure relative to the atmosphere. Airflow into the lungs follows. This is followed by passive exhalation and CO_2 excretion. Or, in nontechnical terms, breathing. Cervical nerves three, four, and five keep you alive. This was the mnemonic every medical student learned.

The third, fourth, and fifth cervical nerves leave the spinal cord on the left and right sides to form the left and right phrenic nerves in the neck. These nerves descend through the thorax and connect to the left and right hemidiaphragms, respectively. Because Philip's tumor was high in the cervical spine above the level of the nerves connected to the phrenics, it was clear that his diaphragmatic dysfunction would remain forever.

Philip was connected to a ventilator. This lifesaving device was connected to Philip's breathing tube that remained in his windpipe. With time, it became evident that Philip would remain dependent on the ventilator at least part of the day to breathe. Long-term ventilator dependence for most means lifelong care in a nursing home. This would almost inevitably lead to a shortened life due to death from pneumonia, wounds from decubitus ulcers (bedsores), or urinary tract infections.

As it was clear that daytime weaning from the ventilator would be a long process, the decision was made within days to perform a tracheostomy. Otorhinolaryngology (ear, nose, and throat) specialists made an incision in his windpipe for placement of a smaller breathing tube that was positioned below his vocal cords to preserve speech. Once Philip had undergone the tracheostomy, we would once again try to wean Philip off the ventilator during the day.

It was obvious that Philip would need long-term ventilatory support. However, it was unclear whether at some point he could be weaned successfully and breathe on his own for part of the day. An initial weaning trial after surgery led to immediate failure. Philip was given the opportunity to breathe on his own, but he could not. He was awake and his breathing center in the brain stem was intact, but the signal from his brain stem came to a stop at the level of the cervical spine where his tumor had grown. The phrenic nerves could not transmit the electrical impulses anxiously awaited by the hemidiaphragms for rhythmic contraction. Without impulse-conducting phrenic nerves, the hemidiaphragms were useless.

In the absence of functioning hemidiaphragms, Philip could not breathe—adequately deliver oxygen or excrete carbon dioxide—without ventilatory support. At the bedside, this manifested as a rapid respiratory rate and a paradoxical breathing pattern as his accessory neck muscles worked furiously to suck in air, but they could not compensate for a lack of diaphragmatic function. This paradoxical breathing pattern reflected ascent of the hemidiaphragms into the thorax rather than contraction downward into the abdomen as is the case with normal, unlabored breathing.

Philip was clearly experiencing air hunger, the uncomfortable sensation of not being able to suck in enough oxygen and excrete carbon dioxide. His weaning trial was quickly stopped, and full ventilatory support was resumed. Tom and Ellen prayed that Philip would be liberated from daytime mechanical ventilation, but they had come to accept that the use of a ventilator during sleep was permanent. They hoped for some degree of independence with a sip-and-puff motorized wheelchair that would eventually enable Philip to cruise around the home on his own.

With their deeply held Christian beliefs, they turned to their church for help. It was a beautiful sunny day in June when Tom met Joseph, a missionary dedicated to the life and work of Padre Pio of Pietrelcina, Italy, who had been beatified and canonized by Pope John II. Padre Pio has a large worldwide following of believers in his ability to heal. Tom escorted Joseph to Philip's bedside. Following prayers, Joseph placed a fingerless glove on Philip's chest to help him breathe once again. At that moment, Ellen was at work and to this day recalls the scent of beautiful flowers that no one else in her environment could smell.

The following day, Philip began to tolerate periods off the ventilator. He was weaning! Was it a miracle, renewed optimism on Philip's part, or just a coincidence? Ellen and Tom have no doubt that this transformative event was nothing short of a miracle. Philip progressively weaned from daytime mechanical ventilation. After three months of hospitalization, he was ready for transfer to a rehab facility.

Philip was usually alert and generally quite comfortable. He quickly and courageously accepted his situation. His dedicated family gave up all personal pursuits in order to care for Philip twenty-four hours a day, seven days a week. By now, he was gaining strength in the accessory muscles of breathing in his neck. His neck muscles were unaffected by the spinal cord injury as innervation of these muscles was from a higher neurological level.

It took months to wean Philip off daytime ventilatory support. This allowed for placement of a cap on his tracheostomy for speech. Nocturnal ventilatory support continued while Philip slept. During sleep, and specifically during REM sleep with its attendant skeletal muscle paralysis, effective breathing relies on intact hemidiaphragm function. Because Philip no longer had functioning hemidiaphragms, there was never any hope that he would be weaned off nighttime ventilatory support.

Philip was transferred to a rehabilitation center as plans for his ultimate disposition were discussed. Philip's family made it clear that there was only one option. Philip would return home once rehabilitation had been completed. A nursing home was never a consideration.

While in rehab, as Philip continued to work with physical therapists in preparation for his return home, Tom and Ellen faced a dilemma. Their two-story town house was not equipped to accommodate Philip's disability. They searched for a home and found a one-level rancher on the market that could be modified to meet Philip's needs so he would be able to access all rooms with his sip-and-puff motorized wheelchair. Philip was becoming skilled at maneuvering his mechanical chariot. With various combinations of sips and puffs controlled by his intact mouth muscles, he would be able to cruise independently to and from any room in the new rancher.

Tom and Ellen were of modest means and were unable to afford the rancher, its modifications, twenty-four-hour nursing, and medical supplies without help. Many in the community showed great compassion and generosity. A childhood friend showed up with a check for $2,000 to pay for a Hoyer lift needed to hoist Philip out of bed. Philip's sister, Cindy, moved in to contribute to housing costs and help with medical care, and a plan was in place for Philip's sister to inherit the home and take over care from Philip's parents if they predeceased him. Other siblings stopped by to help when they could although they were busy with their own families.

One nurse, the owner of a home health agency, ensured that Philip always had nursing coverage and even, when necessary, would pick up a shift herself. Their state representative brought a team of administrators into the home to coordinate insurance coverage. Fortunately, prior to Philip's hospitalization, he had selected the most expensive insurance plan that included a maximum million dollars per year coverage. Without this coverage, Philip's care in the home would have been impossible. He ultimately would have ended up in a facility less equipped to handle his daily needs.

Philip eventually transitioned to healthcare coverage with Medicare and Medicaid. After three months in the hospital, followed by three months in rehab, Philip was ready to come home. Not to his prior town house but to his newly renovated rancher with wheelchair accessibility made possible by the generosity of many in the community. Tom's many friends with valuable skills in home building and construction had volunteered their time on evenings and weekends to make Philip's ranch-style home wheelchair accessible. The home was reconfigured with the sole intention of caring for Philip twenty-four hours a day, seven days a week.

Philip adapted quickly to his new home. Although he had developed many friendships with other disabled souls in rehab, he longed to return to a new normalcy, one where he could watch television, cruise from room-to-room, and join his family for meals. The first years at home were very challenging for Tom and Ellen. Although they had planned well, this was a new situation they faced, and all hardships could not be anticipated.

Lifting Philip was a challenge that required two people. After three years, it became evident that in addition to nursing care, based on Philip's weight, he qualified for a home health aide. As Tom and Ellen aged, they could no longer lift their 200-pound quadriplegic son. Day-to-day life was a learning process for family and healthcare providers alike. As Philip's needs changed, his parents had to adapt and work in the context of the healthcare delivery system to provide for Philip.

The Greatest Virtue: Compassion

Philip intermittently expressed extreme anger after surgery. His loss of the ability to perform activities of daily living, coupled with loss of dignity related to personal hygiene and a total dependence on others, was emotionally painful. However, with the passage of time, he adjusted and adapted to his new existence. Although there were hard days to be sure, Philip became content with his lot in life, a life still filled with the joy of a kind and compassionate family, his ability to speak, hear, see, enjoy food, and control a motorized wheelchair.

Of course, the family alone could not provide all the necessary care for Philip. It was a great effort on the part of nurses, respiratory therapists, wound management clinicians, and other physicians to treat Philip's multiple problems related to quadriplegia. The primary problems that could lead to life-threatening deteriorations included recurrent bouts of sepsis from decubitus ulcers, recurrent pneumonia, and recurrent urinary tract infections.

Everyone loved Philip. Perhaps it was because of his circumstance in combination with his easygoing personality and awesome family that made it so easy to provide Philip everything we could offer.

One of the major problems was convincing Philip's insurance company to cover this costly endeavor. As Philip's family and dedicated nursing staff became so adept at providing his care, subsequent hospitalizations were infrequent. Philip never enjoyed going to the hospital and, in fact, one could argue that he got better care at home from those who knew him well. Most of the treatment he needed was available in the home. Reasons for admissions to the hospital included performance of drainage procedures to remove infected wound collections and to provide medications and fluids for blood pressure support during bouts of sepsis.

One day at work, I received a frantic call from Philip's father. I interrupted my evaluation of another patient because I was concerned that perhaps Philip was having a life-threatening crisis. In fact, Philip felt fine. The crisis was financial. The insurance company was threatening to cut back nursing coverage. This clearly spelled disaster. A decrease in nursing care would undoubtedly increase the chance of multiple hospitalizations and premature death.

Tom picked me up at the hospital and together we met with a panel of insurance executives. I knew that the outcome of this meeting would determine Philip's fate. Philip could not survive in his home without the necessary nursing coverage. He needed frequent attention to all the bodily functions we take for granted as healthy, able individuals. Constant skin care and frequent turning were of paramount importance to prevent skin breakdown and wound infections leading to deadly sepsis.

The meeting was held on the twenty-fifth floor of a Center City corporate office building. Tom and I sat together on one side of a long rectangular table. After a few minutes, a committee of six executives entered the room and sat across the table from us. I had rehearsed my speech, knowing how important it was to convince this committee that Philip's life depended on their financial support. I reviewed Philip's health issues for the group. I knew that I had to appeal to both their pocketbooks and their emotions. I begged them not to cut Philip's nursing coverage and I cautioned them that to do so would ultimately lead to very costly ICU admissions.

Then I told them that Philip's father, Tom, had devoted his entire career as a fireman to saving lives. I asked the committee what they would want if they were in Tom's position and if it were their child at home, quadriplegic, on a ventilator. As I finished my speech, I heard a man weeping. I turned to my right and saw that Philip's dad, this large man who could have played middle linebacker in the NFL, was sobbing. It had finally hit Tom that his son was quadriplegic and would never walk again. The son Tom raised would never father children or enjoy the daily pleasures of life we all take for granted. Philip and his family were at the mercy of this insurance company as it made financial decisions about the fate of their son.

As Tom and I left the insurance company building, we felt optimistic that we had made our case. We were, however, realistic in that we were up against a big business known, or at least perceived, to focus more on the bottom line than humanity. That was not the case this time. Within seventy-two hours, as promised, Tom got a call that nursing coverage would not be cut.

Over the next twenty-five years, I never saw Tom cry again. His family and I remained devoted to Philip and continued to care for him along with a dedicated staff of nurses and respiratory therapists. Over the twenty-five-plus years I cared for Philip, I have been humbled by the great courage, love, and compassion of a family who sacrificed so much and never stopped caring for their son.

Philip's primary medical complications of recurrent infection continued to be problematic. However, with the advent of a specialized suction catheter that allows access to more bronchial breathing tubes, Philip had not suffered from pneumonia; nor had he required fiberoptic bronchoscopy to clear his airways for many years. With great attention to bladder emptying, urinary catheterization, a diverting colostomy, and initiation of a brief course of broad-spectrum antibiotics at the earliest sign of infection, Philip was treated in the home with infrequent hospitalizations.

In recent years, Philip's primary problems had been infection from pressure sores and deep wounds requiring abscess drainage. As a quadriplegic, despite the best efforts to turn him frequently, pressure on his skin remained a major challenge. The skin is a vital organ that separates our internal structures from hostile bacteria on the surface of the skin. With skin breakdown, bacteria invade, multiply, and destroy deeper tissues. Abscess formation leads to dissemination of virulent bacteria into the bloodstream.

This process may culminate in deadly septic shock. Philip had multiple bouts of septic shock related to these incurable, deep-seated bacterial collections. I worried that ultimately Philip would develop a deep wound infection with resistant bacteria leading to refractory septic shock, cardiovascular collapse, and death.

After more than twenty-five years as Philip's physician, I marveled at his extreme courage as he faced the daily challenges of loss of mobility, dignity, and intimacy and was able to find meaning and purpose through close relationships with parents, siblings, nieces, nephews, healthcare providers, and friends. Philip's parents, siblings, dedicated nursing staff, and respiratory therapists remained constantly at his side in their efforts to help him get through each day with unending love and the ultimate virtue: compassion.

Philip never talked about dying. When necessary, he reluctantly agreed to hospitalization for management of life-threatening infections. During hospitalizations, he always expressed interest in returning home as soon as possible. It was evident, though, that after a journey starting in 1992, just two years after President George H. W. Bush signed into law the milestone Americans with Disabilities Act, Philip's condition had declined. The frequency of life-threatening infections had increased and the risk of death had become more looming. Philip's priority was to avoid suffering. He was at peace in his belief that he would one day be with God in heaven.

It was a bitter cold, but bright sunny Sunday in February. Philip's blood pressure was dropping. Certainly, he was experiencing another bout of sepsis from a deep-seated wound infection that was leaking deadly bacteria into his bloodstream. Another trip to the hospital was urgently needed for a drainage procedure by interventional radiology. Although we knew the infection would never be cured, another temporary fix could likely be accomplished. Philip had been through this type of deterioration so many times but the frequency was increasing. After another discussion with Philip regarding his goals, priorities, and what was an acceptable quality of life, he made it clear that the burden/benefit ratio for him had changed.

He no longer wanted to leave his home where he was constantly surrounded by loved ones. It was during the COVID-19 pandemic of 2020. Hospitalization meant days of isolation without family members. Philip and his parents were clearly aware of the ramifications of his decision. Without hospitalization, he would not survive very long. After living as a quadriplegic for twenty-nine years, with awareness of his limited chance of survival, he had become content to live his remaining days at home, supported by his family and nurses. Although I speak of his years of survival, it must be said that he hadn't just survived, he thrived, he enjoyed, he loved, and was loved. He lived a life filled with meaning and purpose by showing so many how to face great adversity with courage and strength. He helped so many to nurture compassion, kindness, empathy, and love.

As the next several days passed, Philip became unresponsive. Although morphine and Ativan were available to relieve pain, breathlessness, and anxiety, it never became necessary. As the bacteria continued to multiply exponentially and invade through the bloodstream, his bodily organs continued to fail. His urine flow stopped as his kidneys no longer functioned. His blood pressure continued to plummet as his heart cells could no longer work in synchrony to squeeze oxygen-carrying blood cells to his vital organs.

At 3:45 A.M., three days after Philip's blood pressure began to deteriorate, Tom was awakened by an alarm signaling Philip's last heartbeat. A heart that had contracted for fifty-eight years no longer functioned. When EMS arrived, they confirmed that Philip had passed away. The ventilator that had pumped oxygen into Philip's lungs for twenty-nine years was no longer able to sustain life. The mechanical sounds of his breathing apparatus could still be heard but were of no value. Without a beating, contracting heart, oxygen delivery was no longer possible. The ventilator was turned off.

I had the great honor of delivering Philip's eulogy. I recounted the life of a courageous soul who lived half of his life on a ventilator—a life many could not fathom nor accept. Yet it was because of a loving compassionate family who sacrificed so much that Philip found twenty-nine years on a ventilator as a quadriplegic well worth the journey. And I am blessed to have known Philip and his family, to have been his doctor and friend, and to have learned so much from all of them all these years.

10

Nicotine Addiction and
Its Devastating Toll

She inhaled her first cigarette at age fourteen behind the
high school gym. As an introvert, Eleanor wanted to fit
in with the cool and popular girls. Addiction to nicotine came
quickly, long before her decision-making frontal lobe was fully
developed. Before she acquired adult judgment, her actions
got her into trouble in school and at home.

As she aged and matured, Eleanor grew up but her
addiction to nicotine continued unabated. Eleanor became an
accountant. She loved numbers and working alone. During the
tax season, it was not uncommon for her to work 100 hours per
week as she plowed through individual tax returns. Though
her business thrived, her personal life stagnated. She preferred
watching television at home in the company of her cat. She
rarely ventured outside her apartment. By the age of fifty-four,
Eleanor had reached a dubious milestone—she smoked two
packs of cigarettes per day for forty years (80 pack years).
Despite the magnitude of her addiction, she never developed
any smoking-related health issues until that year.

I was asked by her primary care physician to evaluate
Eleanor in consultation. When we first met, her deep and
gravelly voice, discolored fingers, and scent of cigarettes were
clues to her underlying nicotine addiction. I suspected the new
onset of shortness of breath she described was in some way
related. After obtaining a detailed history of her symptoms,
it was clear that in recent months her exercise tolerance had
diminished greatly. A walk to the corner drugstore for a carton
of cigarettes became a challenge. Because her addiction was

so strong, she pushed through with a slow-paced walk while frequently stopping to catch her breath.

A physical exam that day revealed two major findings. With the use of my stethoscope, a clinical tool developed by French physician René Laënnec in 1816 and still of great clinical value more than two centuries later, it was evident that Eleanor's breath sounds were abnormal. One of the beauties of birth with two lungs is that physicians can listen during auscultation of the chest for any differences. Eleanor's right lung sounded quite normal. With each inhalation and exhalation, I could easily appreciate breath sounds as her bronchus filled the tiny air sacs in her right lung with air. As she exhaled, no wheezes, often detected in smokers, were evident.

When I gently placed my stethoscope over the left hemithorax (left side of her chest), however, I listened intently but heard nothing as she was breathing in and out. Air entry through the left main stem bronchus (that extends into her lung) was undetectable. This likely meant one of two things. Either her left main stem bronchus was blocked by a cancer or fluid had accumulated in her left hemithorax to such a great degree that it was squishing down her left lung thereby preventing air entry.

This fluid accumulation in the pleural space is known as a pleural effusion. A layer of thin, Saran Wrap–like tissue covers the surface of the entire lung. Another similar thin layer of tissue lines the inside of the chest wall. Normally, minimal fluid between these two layers serves as a lubricant to allow the lungs to inflate and deflate without rubbing.

When I examined Eleanor's fingers, I noted pink nail beds consistent with normal oxygenation. However, all of her fingertips demonstrated spongy enlargement, known as clubbing. This prominent finding in the context of Eleanor's history of cigarette smoking strongly suggested the presence of a lung cancer. Eleanor asked, "So what do you think is happening?" I shared with her my concerns about fluid accumulation or a blockage. I ordered a chest X-ray to determine which of these two possibilities explained her clinical presentation.

Eleanor asked me how we would proceed with each of those scenarios. We discussed that if there were a blockage, I would perform a fiberoptic bronchoscopy to evaluate the inside of her airways. If it were fluid, I would drain it from her chest. I knew that in either case, the likelihood of a good outcome was small. If a large amount of fluid had accumulated, it would likely return after drainage. If there were a blockage, it would likely be an incurable lung cancer secondary to many years of cigarette smoking.

After review of the chest X-ray, which confirmed the presence of a large pleural effusion, I scheduled Eleanor for an outpatient thoracentesis to drain the fluid.

We met at 9:00 A.M. the following day in our outpatient procedure unit. After I obtained written consent, Eleanor rested in a sitting position with her arms atop two pillows placed comfortably on a patient meal table. I began to localize my point of entry into her left hemithorax. Mark, the nurse, helped Eleanor stay still and supported her during this relatively painless procedure.

As with many surgical procedures, older physicians teach younger physicians how to safely perform such interventions. You cannot open a textbook and learn to perform a procedure. These skills are passed down from generation to generation. Prior to marking her chest for the spot of fluid removal, I again listened to her lungs to confirm the proper side. Though rare, wrong-side surgery does occur. I reached into my pocket and found a silver dime. After counting down two rib interspaces below the tip of her left scapula, that triangular bone so instrumental in shoulder movement, I firmly pressed the dime onto Eleanor's skin and left a circular target on her back.

I opened a packet of Betadine antiseptic swabs and in a circular movement cleaned the area of the dime indentation as well as a larger surrounding circle approximately three inches in diameter. After numbing the area with local lidocaine, I introduced a needle connected to a vacuum bottle through two feet of tubing and drained 1.5 quarts of dark bloody fluid. Although I was rather convinced that this reflected underlying malignancy, I held out hope that it was a more treatable process such as infection.

Eleanor tolerated the procedure quite well. We met the following day to review the results. The pathology report confirmed the presence of cancer cells. Specific stains strongly suggested lung cancer. My suspicion, unfortunately, had been confirmed.

It was 1995, and, in those days, we had not yet discovered the great advances of driver mutations and immunotherapy that, for some with advanced lung cancer, can greatly prolong life. Based upon known statistics at the time, I knew that Eleanor's prognosis was poor. We discussed the possibility of chemotherapy but, influenced by my pessimism regarding its efficacy at the time, Eleanor declined. When her shortness of breath returned one week later, it was obvious that cancer cells inflaming the pleural surfaces had led to re-accumulation of fluid in the pleural space.

Upon my request and after discussion with Eleanor, a thoracic surgeon placed a chest tube into Eleanor's pleural space to drain the fluid completely. To prevent re-accumulation, the surgeon instilled a chemical known as bleomycin, ordinarily used as a chemotherapy agent. In this situation, it would not have any antineoplastic effect (to attack the cancer) but would serve as a sclerosing agent causing an inflammatory response so the surfaces would stick together and prevent further fluid buildup. I informed Eleanor that this procedure, known as pleurodesis, was only for palliative purposes to decrease shortness of breath and prevent fluid re-accumulation. I told her that it would not halt the progression of her underlying lung cancer.

Eleanor was able to return to work. She found comfort in the numbers of accounting. It allowed her to forget that she was dying of cancer. It also allowed her to avoid the inevitable truth that she was likely to die alone. Eleanor had never married and had no children. She was estranged from her brother who lived in Seattle, and her parents were deceased. When Eleanor returned to see me in the office three months later, it was evident that she had lost considerable weight. Cancer cachexia (weakness and wasting) had robbed her of her appetite. Eleanor was now very thin appearing and with decrease in the soft tissue of her face, her cheekbones had become very prominent.

Although the shortness of breath never returned, Eleanor noted new onset of hip pain and difficulty ambulating without a cane. She knew she was dying. A scan obtained that afternoon showed that her cancer had spread to multiple bones, including her hips, spine, and ribs. Eleanor returned the following day for the discussion that many physicians unfortunately tend to avoid, a vital discussion that, if not performed, deprives patients of important decision making while they feel well enough to express their goals, priorities, and personal choices about how they wish to spend their remaining days of life.

Because Eleanor was extremely bright and insightful, I did not have much to explain. When I told Eleanor that the cancer had spread into her bones, she nodded and said she understood. What she and I both understood at that moment was that an addiction to nicotine from an early age had caused a proliferating cancer to disseminate wildly and widely throughout her body, causing pain and suffering as her final days approached. I nodded when she expressed the shame she felt about her inability to quit smoking for a sustained period of time. She began to cry. She disclosed to me that nonsmokers do not understand brain chemistry and the overwhelming power of nicotine addiction. She recounted the many times she tried to stop and the many medications that failed to lead to sustained smoking cessation.

I agreed and acknowledged the pain and her feelings of shame. For the first time, I grasped her hand as we outlined a plan for her future. I reassured her that we would minimize her suffering with morphine, a narcotic; Ativan, a benzodiazepine antianxiety medicine; and if needed, oxygen supplementation. I recommended that home hospice pay her a visit soon. We discussed end-of-life issues including resuscitation efforts such as cardiopulmonary resuscitation and mechanical ventilation.

Although as a physician I felt no obligation to offer futile care, certainly Eleanor had the right to engage in the discussion of end-of-life care, including life support. Her notion of futility may differ from mine. Although the decision and process of withholding ventilatory support is generally less burdensome than withdrawal of life support, the patient has a right to be involved in the decision-making process.

After gaining an understanding of Eleanor's priorities and goals, I advised against initiation of mechanical ventilation or chest compression should her lungs or heart cease to function. I shared with her that in my experience these interventions for her at this point in life would not be appropriate and likely would cause additional suffering. Certainly, I respected her autonomy as a competent adult and her right to decide which interventions should be provided and which should be withheld. However, I felt compelled to share my advice in the context of Eleanor's disease trajectory, likelihood of survival, and my years of experience managing patients at the end stages of life.

Eleanor agreed and made it clear that her top priority was comfort. We concurred that she would be designated Do Not Resuscitate/Do Not Intubate. A team of hospice nurses arrived at Eleanor's home the next day. These wonderfully compassionate providers, who have dedicated their lives to walking patients down the path of their final days, were there to deliver physical, emotional, and spiritual support. As pain progressed, and intermittent oral morphine became necessary more frequently, Eleanor requested admission to inpatient hospice for care in her final days.

During her last days of life, Eleanor lapsed in and out of consciousness on a morphine infusion. Her only human contact consisted of brief nursing checks to ensure adequate pain control. Her periods of alertness were progressively shortened. What were her conscious thoughts during these brief lucid moments as she surveyed the barren walls with feelings of isolation? Did she lament that no loved ones were present to comfort her? Did she regret not reconciling with her estranged brother as I had advised? Did fleeting memories of a shortened life surface to consciousness?

In the final hours, Eleanor entered a deep state of unconsciousness. Verbal and tactile stimulation by the nursing staff elicited no meaningful response. The morphine infusion continued at a steady rate and maintained her in a state of comfort by all outward appearances. Although impossible to know with certainty whether she was experiencing physical or emotional discomfort, no signs of distress were evident. In the final hours of her life, her breathing patterns changed significantly. Prolonged periods exceeding one to two minutes of absent respiratory effort were punctuated by deep gasps: her brain's feeble attempts to suck in just one more breath, one more drop of life. With each breath, a rattling sound could be heard in the hallway as air passed through oral secretions that Eleanor could no longer swallow.

Death was imminent. The timeline of Eleanor's first gasp as a newborn to her last gasp as an adult was soon to be completed. Nobody witnessed Eleanor's final effort to breathe. The time of death, an estimate at best, was recorded as 1:35 A.M. after the medical resident listened with her stethoscope for any remnant of life. Minutes after her last breath of air, her heart, deprived of oxygen, stopped beating. A heart that had contracted rhythmically for more than fifty years no longer served its purpose. A heart that ensured the delivery of oxygen to all her body's cells no longer functioned. This miraculous four-chambered pump, along with all of Eleanor's bodily organs, no longer shared life's greatest gift nor grasped its ultimate mystery: the mystery of the human body with its organs functioning as a great symphony. The music was now silent. A masterpiece of a human life ending with a brief decrescendo of breaths had finished with a quiet ending.

———————

The process of informed consent is bidirectional, between physician and patient. Prior to suggesting a course of action such as withholding or withdrawing life support, the physician must have a clear up-to-date understanding of the patient's medical condition as well as the prevailing standard of care for treating such a condition. This often requires consultation with colleagues who may have special expertise in the management of such a disease process.

With medical information platforms such as UpToDate, access to new developments in treatment along with the likelihood of benefit and harm is more readily available than ever before in the long history of the practice of medicine. It is only through advancement of the physician's knowledge base that she or he is well positioned to suggest a course of action consistent with the patient's goals and priorities. In the absence of such knowledge, valid informed consent is not possible.

Since 1964, when Luther Terry, Surgeon General of the United States Public Health Service, concluded that cigarette smoking is a cause of lung cancer, many advances in early detection and treatment have helped diminish the great suffering caused by this poisonous tobacco product:

- Targeted therapy in patients with specific driver mutations, immunotherapy, and chemotherapy can prolong survival in patients with Stage IV metastatic non-small cell lung cancer.

- Early palliative care consultation can improve quality of life and decrease futile end-of-life care in patients with Stage IV metastatic non-small cell lung cancer.

- Low-dose CT scanning for early lung cancer detection, an imaging technique published in the *New England Journal of Medicine* in 2011 after a study of 53,000 patients with high risk for lung cancer, has helped the United States Preventive Services Task Force establish recommendations in an effort to decrease lung cancer mortality. An update in March 2021, indicated that candidates include those with:

  - Twenty-pack years' smoking history (one pack per day for twenty years equals twenty-pack years)

  - An age of fifty to eighty

  - Patients who smoked within the past fifteen years. These recommendations may change with time. The reader is referred to the Centers for Disease Control guidelines for the most recent recommendations.

- Smoking cessation clinics and medications such as nicotine replacement therapy and varenicline are available to assist patients in the process.

Unfortunately, despite these advances, according to the federal government's Centers for Disease Control and Prevention (CDC), millions of Americans continue to smoke and 438,000 Americans die each year prematurely from cigarette smoking. Lung cancer remains a common cause of cancer deaths worldwide.

I often think of Eleanor and the many other patients who have suffered greatly from the effects of nicotine addiction brought on by cigarette smoking. As a pulmonologist, I have witnessed great misery from devastating physical harm caused by years of inhaling tars and nicotine contained in cigarettes. Certainly, use of tobacco products tops the list worldwide as the number one cause of preventable death and contributes to considerable breathlessness as well as physical and emotional suffering.

11

No Tube

Fred was an auto mechanic with more work than he could handle. He rarely took a day off from work. When he presented to the emergency department with progressive shortness of breath, it took considerable effort to convince him that he needed to be admitted for further treatment of his COPD exacerbation.

Fred had smoked cigarettes since the age of twelve. Despite multiple attempts to quit, he continued to inhale two packs a day. Years of inhaling from these deadly white paper cylinders filled with tobacco had caused considerable damage to his lungs. He developed emphysema, a form of chronic obstructive pulmonary disease. His condition made him quite vulnerable to respiratory tract infections leading to transient and life-threatening declines in lung function.

When Fred was evaluated in the hospital, he appeared to be in mild respiratory distress. His respiratory rate was elevated at twenty-four breaths per minute to compensate for his diminished pulmonary function. His oxygen level was below normal. His carbon dioxide was elevated. These two findings in conjunction with an elevated respiratory rate spelled potential disaster if not appropriately treated.

Unfortunately, COPD exacerbations have become a very common cause of hospitalizations nationwide. It is almost always caused by smoking cigarettes and has become one of the leading causes of death worldwide. Although COPD exacerbations are usually successfully treated leading to a return to baseline function, ongoing smoking would certainly cause progression of Fred's lung disease, ultimately leading to profound disability and death.

Fred was admitted to the intermediate critical care unit. In addition to inhalational therapy with medicines to dilate his bronchial tubes, he was given intravenous steroids to shrink the inflammation that contributed to airway narrowing. Fred also was placed on a mask with a noninvasive ventilator device to assist him in his breathing by delivering oxygen and removing carbon dioxide from his lungs.

Initially, Fred showed clinical improvement. His oxygen and CO2 levels were closer to baseline and his breathing became less labored. That all changed one afternoon when Fred's nurse noted that he was blue, agitated, and breathing very rapidly. The rapid response team was summoned and within minutes a team of physicians, nurses, and respiratory therapists was at his bedside. A STAT arterial blood gas revealed that the carbon dioxide level circulating in his blood was two times the normal level. This indicated that Fred had developed worsening respiratory failure and would require placement of a breathing tube in his windpipe for attachment to a mechanical ventilator to breathe for him more effectively until his COPD exacerbation resolved.

I heard a page over the hospital speaker system, "Anesthesia STAT." This emergency declaration always causes a visceral response as a patient somewhere in the hospital is close to death. When anesthesia arrived at the bedside, I explained to Fred that a breathing tube would be placed in his windpipe so he could breathe more easily. I reviewed with Fred that he would be sedated and given other medicines to keep him comfortable while the machine relieved his breathlessness. Once the endotracheal tube was secured, he would then be carefully moved to the intensive care unit for close monitoring and treatment.

After an initial period of calm, Fred began screaming, "No tube. No tube." He repeatedly removed his noninvasive ventilator mask. The pulse oximeter alarm was sounding, and the dropping oxygen level raised a red flag that he was minutes away from death. As his oxygen level declined, and his carbon dioxide level continued to rise, it was clear that at any minute his heart rate would drop, and he would have a cardiac arrest.

When the heart muscle is deprived of oxygen, the heart rate gradually "bradys down" or decreases and then stops.

Of course, we wanted to avoid such a catastrophe. We had a dilemma. Did Fred have the right to refuse placement of a breathing tube? Did he have the capacity to make such an important decision? There was no time to confer with his wife or convene the Ethics Committee or consult with Legal Affairs. His heart could stop at any minute with death soon to follow. Certainly, every human has the privilege of autonomy. Every competent adult has the right to refuse various forms of therapy based upon personal or religious beliefs and goals. If we followed Fred's instructions, his life would soon end. Did we have the right to ignore his declaration of "no tube" and if we did, would we be guilty of assault?

Although Fred had COPD, he did not have a terminal illness. The overwhelming likelihood was that we could intervene by temporarily supporting Fred's failing lungs and usher him back to his baseline functioning, perhaps within a week or two. The attending anesthesiologist turned to me and asked for guidance. Without hesitating, I declared, "intubate." It was evident that Fred was agitated, hypoxic (oxygen deprived), and hypercapnic (excessive carbon dioxide) and, therefore, did not have the capacity to make a life-and-death decision.

I acted on the premise of implied consent. There was no evidence in his medical record that he had previously expressed a wish to withhold ventilatory support should the need arise. I opted for life. Implied consent assumes what a mentally competent person would want in similar life-and-death situations. Although I did not know this patient, and though it was my responsibility to honor the concept of autonomy, I also was obliged to make a decision where the patient lacked the capacity to make his own decision.

A sedating medication was infused through the intravenous line in Fred's arm. The Ambu Bag, used for artificial respiration, was placed over his face and rhythmically squeezed by the respiratory therapist. As 100 percent oxygen was being pushed into his diseased lungs, his oxygen level began to rise to a safer level, allowing the anesthesia specialists to proceed with placing a curved plastic tube through his mouth, past his vocal cords, and into his windpipe. At the end of the breathing tube was a small cuff that was inflated once the tube was in position. This inflated cuff secured the tube in place and prevented air from leaking around the breathing tube.

After three days of care in the intensive care unit on the ventilator, Fred's sedation was stopped. His lung function had improved significantly. An arterial blood gas showed normalization of his oxygen and carbon dioxide levels. He was given a spontaneous breathing trial where ventilatory support was minimized as most of the breathing was through his own effort. After a successful spontaneous breathing trial, the breathing tube was removed.

That evening, Fred was sitting up in a chair, chatting with his wife and young children. His voice was a bit hoarse from the irritating breathing tube rubbing up against his vocal cords. Otherwise, Fred felt great. He denied any breathlessness. On the day of discharge from the hospital, he thanked the team for the care he had received and pledged to quit smoking. He was provided with detailed information to assist him with smoking cessation. When I asked Fred about his experience that fateful afternoon when he was close to death, Fred replied that he could not remember much but did recall a young female doctor holding his hand and appearing extremely concerned.

Autonomy is a core value in modern American civilization. Its Greek origin describes an opportunity to act independently and in accordance with one's values and priorities. According to the American Medical Association Code of Medical Ethics, "A patient with decision-making capacity has the right to decline any medical intervention or ask that an intervention be stopped even when the decision is expected to lead to death regardless of whether or not the individual was terminally ill."

In the context of medical decision making, autonomy is fulfilled through the process of informed consent. Every individual has the ongoing right to determine and choose which recommended intervention will and will not be performed. Although it is assumed that a physician's recommendation regarding a treatment, intervention, or procedure is provided with the patient's best interest at heart, the ultimate decision rests with the informed and consenting individual.

At the moment informed consent is obtained, however, the physician must determine with reasonable certainty whether the patient possesses the capacity to make such a decision. Such a judgment must never be taken lightly as the ramifications for the patient may be profound and life altering. To determine a patient's capacity for medical decision making, cognitive functioning must be adequately assessed. Various chronic medical disorders such as psychiatric illness or degenerative neurological diseases may sufficiently impair cognition so as to render a patient incapable of making an informed decision. Additionally, hospitalized patients often endure temporary alterations in cognitive functioning from metabolic disturbances, infection, or medications. It is incumbent upon the physician to recognize these potentially reversible effects and intervene to correct these perturbations as able.

Dr. Jason Karlawish and Dr. James Lai have developed a framework to assist the medical community in assessing a patient's capacity for medical decision making. Four key elements in this assessment include:

- *Understanding.* After listening to a physician's explanation, the patient should be able to restate the nature of his or her medical condition as well as the intervention, treatment, or procedure proposed.

- *Expression of Choice.* Based upon his or her understanding, the patient should be able to express a decision regarding the proposed treatment, intervention, or procedure.

- *Appreciation.* The patient should be able to explain how the decision will directly impact that patient as an individual as it relates to the potential benefits and harms of the proposed treatment, intervention, or procedure.

- *Reasoning.* The patient should be able to explain the consequences that will occur specifically to that individual if a decision is made by the patient not to proceed with the recommended treatment, intervention, or procedure.

Clearly, the physician's explanation and choice of words must be consistent with the patient's level of education and familiarity with medical jargon. A patient with an eighth-grade level of education will require a different explanation than a patient who is a nurse or physician possessing greater understanding and medical knowledge.

If it is the judgment of the physician that the patient has sufficient cognitive impairment causing lack of capacity to contribute to a medical decision-making process to fulfill informed consent, then a surrogate decision maker, if time allows, must be sought. Ideally, this substitute would be one previously designated in writing by the patient.

Unfortunately, in the day-to-day practice of critical care medicine, such designations often have not been established in advance. In such a case, and consistent with prevailing state laws, a hierarchy of individuals is pursued to decide on the patient's behalf, with the patient's best interest at heart, and preferably as previously articulated by that patient at a time of better health and cognition. Generally, the order of authority is spouse, adult child, parent, siblings. For acceptable surrogate decision making, the physician will want to ensure that the surrogate indeed has capacity at that moment and is acting in the best interest of the patient. These issues can add layers of challenge that might require hospital legal counsel.

In time-sensitive situations, however, where an intervention is emergently required to prevent death or disability, a physician may act based upon implied consent rather than informed consent. This alternative form of consent assumes the following:

- The patient lacks capacity to provide informed consent at that moment in time.

- An emergent intervention is necessary to prevent death or disability.

- A reasonable individual with capacity would agree to such an intervention.

- The physician is acting in the patient's best interest.

- There is insufficient time to obtain consent from a surrogate and a delay would likely cause substantial harm or death to the patient.

It is clearly evident that all of these conditions were met when, despite Fred's proclamation of "no tube," an endotracheal tube placement was emergently needed for mechanical ventilation to sustain life. Although the patient with capacity has the right to choose an option that a physician might not have selected, one must always protect the patient lacking capacity from making a "bad" decision that a physician reasonably believed the patient would not have made if the patient had capacity at that moment to make a decision.

12

Acute Respiratory Distress Syndrome

It was 6:00 P.M. and my day's work was finished. I headed to my car in the hospital parking garage. I looked forward to joining my family for dinner. My cell phone rang and the emergency department attending physician asked if I were still in the hospital. After sixty seconds of conversation, I responded, "I will meet you in five minutes." Dinner would have to wait. During my brisk walk to the emergency department, I called my wife and told her to start dinner with the children without me.

When I arrived at the emergency department, the clerk guided me to cubicle number 4. Mr. Aronson was surrounded by his family and a team of healthcare providers attempting to stabilize his acute medical condition. I introduced myself as a pulmonary/critical care medicine physician and quickly learned that Mr. Aronson was an eighty-year-old man who was in good health, enjoyed independent functioning, and had felt quite well until his recent onset of fevers and a burning sensation with urination.

On exam, he was breathing at a rate of thirty-eight times per minute—twice the normal rate—and was diaphoretic (sweating heavily) and unable to complete full sentences without gasping for breaths. Review of his chest X-ray demonstrated no abnormalities. Why was this elderly gentleman in respiratory distress despite a normal-appearing chest X-ray?

The answer surfaced after review of an arterial blood gas test using a blood sample obtained from his radial artery. He was experiencing a metabolic acidosis due to urosepsis. That

82

is, a severe systemic infection was causing a dangerous buildup of a lactic acid in his bloodstream. To prevent a life-threatening drop in blood pH, his brain stem responded by sending neural messages to his hemidiaphragms to breathe rapidly in an effort to blow off the volatile acid, carbon dioxide. Failure to do so would cause a plummeting blood pH, not compatible with life.

It was obvious that Mr. Aronson was showing signs of fatigue and ventilatory support was urgently needed to assist his feeble attempts to breathe. I explained to Mr. Aronson and his family that treatment of his life-threatening urosepsis required antibiotics, intravenous saline infusions to support a dropping blood pressure, and placement of a breathing tube to diminish his work of breathing.

Although Mr. Aronson was struggling to breathe, he maintained capacity for decision making and declared that he wanted to be treated aggressively. Anesthesia staff placed an endotracheal tube in his windpipe without difficulty. A chest X-ray subsequently revealed that the breathing tube was properly positioned in his trachea and both lungs appeared to be well expanded with no evidence of pneumonia or fluid.

Mr. Aronson's signs of respiratory distress resolved quickly as a mechanical ventilator breathed for him. He was transferred to the intensive care unit and cared for by the night shift team of a medical resident, medical intern, and critical care nurse. I then headed home to find that my family had finished dinner. I grabbed a quick bite and called the ICU resident to review plans for the night for Mr. Aronson and other critically ill patients in the intensive care unit.

The decision to place an endotracheal tube for initiation of mechanical ventilation is often a challenging one and may be divided into five major categories:

- *Airway Maintenance.*
  - Patients with upper airway obstruction due to tumor, foreign body, swelling related to medication, infection, or an allergic reaction.

- Coma with a risk of aspiration in patients with a Glasgow Coma Scale of 8 or less. (A Glasgow Coma Scale is a 15-point scale that evaluates the level of consciousness; a lower score indicates the patient is at greater risk.)

- *Inability to Deliver Oxygen.* As the alveoli become thickened and destroyed through disease processes such as COVID pneumonia or ARDS (Acute Respiratory Distress Syndrome), diffusion of oxygen through these typically porous alveoli may become sufficiently impaired. Prior to placement of a breathing tube for mechanical ventilation, less invasive means aimed at maintaining an oxygen saturation of 92 percent or above are typically attempted and include, in sequential order: low-flow nasal oxygen one–six liters per minute, high-flow nasal oxygen up to sixty liters per minute, and noninvasive ventilation with BiPAP (a bi-level positive airway pressure device).

- *Inability to Excrete Carbon Dioxide.* With various pulmonary disease processes, the mechanics of the lungs are impaired and cannot sufficiently excrete carbon dioxide. Normal blood pH is 7.35–7.45. Extremes of pH are not compatible with life. With inability to excrete the volatile acid, carbon dioxide, the blood pH will drop potentially to life-threatening levels. A common cause in critical care is the exacerbation of chronic obstructive pulmonary disease triggered by a respiratory tract infection. In the tachypneic (breathing rapidly) or lethargic patient, an arterial blood gas is often obtained to measure the blood pH.

  If the blood pH is between 7.25 and 7.35 in the setting of an elevated PCO2, noninvasive ventilation with BiPAP is a lifesaving intervention that may allow avoidance of placement of the more invasive endotracheal tube for mechanical ventilation. Although noninvasive ventilation may be considered with a pH of less than 7.25, the clinician must be equipped and quickly prepared to place an endotracheal tube for mechanical ventilation if improvement based upon follow-up blood gas, respiratory rate, work of breathing, and general patient appearance is not quickly evident.

- *Neuromuscular Weakness.* Guillain-Barré syndrome is the prototypic potentially reversible neuromuscular disease that may require temporary ventilatory support as the ascending paralysis in some patients involves the muscles of respiration. Simple testing at the bedside performed by a respiratory therapist can help assess respiratory muscle strength and guide the physician regarding the decision to initiate mechanical ventilation. The 20-30-40 rule described at the Mayo Clinic involves:

  — *Vital Capacity:* (the total amount of air a patient can breathe out forcibly) less than 20 cc/kg

  — *Maximum Inspiratory Pressure:* (the greatest inspiratory pressure the patient can suck in against a manometer) 30 mmHg

  — *Maximum Expiratory Pressure:* (the greatest pressure a patient can generate during expiration) 40 mmHg

  If any of these three reduced values are met or if there is a trend toward these thresholds, mechanical ventilation should be strongly considered in an effort to prevent a respiratory arrest due to weakness of the breathing muscles. Failure to recognize this window of opportunity to intervene electively with mechanical ventilation may lead to death or permanent disability from hypoxic brain injury.

  Ultimately, there is no substitute for clinical judgment. The placement of an endotracheal tube for mechanical ventilation should strongly be considered if the patient has any of the following symptoms: a sustained respiratory rate exceeding thirty, demonstration of increasing work of breathing manifesting as difficulty speaking full sentences, diaphoresis, use of accessory neck muscles to suck in air, or paradoxical breathing pattern where the chest and abdomen excursions are out of sync with each other.

- *General Anesthesia.* For patients requiring general anesthesia for surgery, placement of an endotracheal tube for mechanical ventilation is necessary as the patient is often rendered paralyzed and dependent on mechanical ventilation for ventilatory support.

When I arrived in the intensive care unit for rounds the following morning, we discussed Mr. Aronson's clinical course first. Although he had been quite stable through the night, I was informed by the sleep-deprived intern, who had slept not a wink, that Mr. Aronson's oxygen level had been gradually declining over the early morning hours.

Review of a 6:00 A.M. chest X-ray demonstrated a dramatic change. Mr. Aronson had developed bilateral fluffy infiltrates, a sign that his alveoli had become flooded with fluid. My hope the night before had been for a quick liberation from mechanical ventilation. That was no longer possible. Despite administration of the diuretic Lasix to increase urination in the hope of removing fluid from his lungs, his oxygenation and follow-up chest X-rays demonstrated continued deterioration.

The pressure required by his ventilator to provide adequate volumes of air was increasing. His lungs were becoming like stiff balloons. Mr. Aronson was developing the greatly feared complication of sepsis known as ARDS (Acute Respiratory Distress Syndrome). His lungs had become a battleground between circulating bacteria from his urinary tract infection and the body's dysfunctional inflammatory response. Release of inflammatory mediators was destroying the delicate interface between the gas-exchanging alveolar surfaces and their surrounding blood vessels. This porous interface normally allows the diffusion of oxygen from alveoli into blood vessels and carbon dioxide from blood vessels into alveoli while maintaining impermeability to fluid from the tiny vessels. Now with millions of tiny holes in the damaged capillary walls, fluid was flooding into Mr. Aronson's air sacs and he was drowning.

Acute Respiratory Distress Syndrome

The disease process of ARDS was initially described to the medical community by Dr. David Ashbaugh in 1967 and later became of increasing interest during the Vietnam War when soldiers who endured horrific trauma developed a non-cardiogenic pulmonary edema characterized by diffuse bilateral flooding of the alveoli evident on chest X-ray. We have since learned that many systemic insults such as pneumonia, aspiration, burns, trauma, pancreatitis, and sepsis can lead to a similar lung injury resulting in flooding of these tiny delicate air sacs due to seeping of fluid from surrounding pulmonary capillaries.

Although the causes may vary, the end result is the release of inflammatory mediators tearing millions of tiny holes in the lining of pulmonary capillary walls and a subsequent deluge. This flooding impairs gas exchange and threatens death if not quickly treated with appropriate ventilatory support and management of the underlying culprit, such as sepsis.

Although mortality for ARDS remains high, a major development in management was published in the *New England Journal of Medicine* in the year 2000. It was definitively demonstrated that providing smaller volumes from the ventilator led to improved survival. What is termed "lung protective strategy" has become the standard of care in the management of patients with ARDS. This has resulted in a substantial decrease in mortality from approximately 40 percent to approximately 30 percent based upon this landmark multicenter study.

Since 1928, when Dr. Philip Drinker and Dr. Louis Agassiz Shaw introduced mechanical ventilators to the world, much research and development have led to more advanced generations of these life support devices. Ventilators can maintain breathing for patients while they suffer from a severe lung insult or undergo general anesthesia for surgery. Their use in the twentieth century peaked during the polio epidemic when viral invasion caused respiratory muscle paralysis and death without ventilatory support.

A peak in the twenty-first century occurred in 2020, when a pandemic raged worldwide. A novel coronavirus that originated in Wuhan, China, known as SARS-CoV-2 was the cause of the disease labeled COVID-19. Like other viruses, such as influenza, it caused a diffuse lung injury leading to ARDS. Because it was a novel virus that our immune systems had never encountered, susceptibility was greatly heightened and mortality dramatically increased.

———————

When I next met with Mr. Aronson's family in the intensive care unit, I remained optimistic but showed concern that his development of ARDS rendered treatment more challenging. His urosepsis was well controlled on antibiotic therapy, his blood pressure no longer required medicines known as pressors, and his oxygen requirement was not excessive. I explained that, although we supported Mr. Aronson with low tidal volume ventilation, nutritional support, and antibiotics, we would patiently await his ability to heal the lung injury that had resulted from sepsis-induced inflammatory mediators. I shared concerns that other problems such as ventilator-associated pneumonia, pulmonary embolism, and GI bleeding could occur and that we would continue in our efforts to prevent them.

We wanted to liberate him from the ventilator as soon as possible to decrease the likelihood of these life-threatening events but not any sooner than his lung healing would allow. Although normally we breathe 21 percent oxygen, Mr. Aronson was requiring 60 percent oxygen to maintain an oxygen saturation of 88 percent, the minimum acceptable level for delivery of oxygen to his tissues. Liberation from mechanical ventilation would have to wait until his oxygen requirement diminished.

Unfortunately, as the days passed, his oxygen requirement increased. By day fourteen, Mr. Aronson was requiring 100 percent oxygen. Despite various manipulations of the ventilator known as salvage techniques, he was dying. High oxygen concentrations required are known to be toxic and contribute to a vicious cycle. His worsening lung injury and fibrosis formation required higher amounts of oxygen. These higher amounts of oxygen caused additional lung injury.

During my last meeting with Mr. Aronson's family, I shared my decreasing optimism. Despite maximal ventilatory support, his oxygen saturation was approaching levels not compatible with life. Mr. Aronson appeared comfortable in a medically induced coma. We focused on efforts to diminish his suffering. The family, however, was suffering greatly. They were about to lose a loved one from progressive refractory respiratory failure. After our discussions, we agreed that should Mr. Aronson's heart stop or his blood pressure drop, no efforts at further resuscitation would follow. These interventions would be futile and only prolong the inevitable.

The determination of medical futility is a challenging process with multiple contributing factors. In the ICU setting, critical care physicians, supported by palliative care providers, guide patients and their surrogates in decision making regarding life support when futility has become evident. As critical illness with multisystem organ failure progresses unabated, and the prospect of recovery to an acceptable quality of life becomes negligible, discussions of withholding or withdrawing life support and a focus on comfort care become necessary.

The discussion, often initiated by the critical care physician, is influenced by clinical experience, conversations with relevant consultants, and knowledge of the medical literature. However, whether consciously or unconsciously, the clinician is influenced by personal beliefs that may be quite different from those of the patient or the patient's surrogate. These differences may influence the ultimate decision as to whether a patient or surrogate agrees with the medical recommendation to withhold or withdraw life support because of medical futility.

Although it is generally agreed upon that a physician is not compelled to provide what she or he deems to be futile care, in reality it would be unusual for life support to be withdrawn against the wishes of a patient or patient's surrogate. In such a situation, ongoing daily discussions include clinical updates, but it is sometimes disease progression that leads to death from cardiovascular collapse while the patient remains on life support. The previously expressed opinion of futility is then confirmed and the breathing tube, no longer sustaining life, is withdrawn.

In the time of a pandemic, such as the one we faced due to COVID-19, limited resources magnify the importance of discussing end-of-life issues. If the need for lifesaving devices exceeds the supply, an objective approach to the allocation of ventilators becomes a necessity. This has led some institutions in the United States to form committees known as COVID triage teams.

These committees, which include critical care providers with no professional or personal relationship with involved patients, might be called upon to apply a detailed point system that takes into account the likelihood of survival and discharge to home. The team might also consider the presence of comorbidities such as incurable malignancy, advanced cardiac disease, and end stage renal disease. The team might need to perform an assessment to determine which of two patients in need of one remaining ventilator would be the recipient. This decision about who shall live and who shall die when life saving equipment is scarce is undoubtedly the most difficult decision one could contemplate in the practice of medicine. Fortunately, in our institution, this type of resource allocation has not become necessary. Other centers within the United States and abroad may be less fortunate.

In December 2020, we were in the second wave of the COVID-19 pandemic and many hospital ICUs were overwhelmed with critically ill patients suffering from ARDS due to COVID pneumonia. If all ventilators in a hospital are being utilized, one could contemplate being called upon to consider the terrifying prospect of removing life support, without consent, from one patient deemed to have minimal chance of survival so that a younger, healthier, critically ill patient might be given a chance of living. However, this unsettling prospect raises many ethical and legal hurdles that would certainly challenge such an extreme intervention.

I left the hospital that day with a feeling of great sadness. Although I cherish the great moments of lifesaving interventions I had witnessed over four decades, I mourn the loss of patients who have died in our ICU on my watch, and I forever wonder whether we could have done more for those who did not survive. I also mourn the loss of thousands of others who have died in ICUs throughout the world.

I also often think about the many patients who survived critical illness only to be left with long-standing disability with weakness, breathlessness, and in many cases, post-traumatic stress disorder. For many who were successfully liberated from mechanical ventilation and survived a critical illness, a long journey awaited them. Dedicated physical therapists, occupational therapists, speech therapists, mental health workers, and pulmonary physicians assist them in achieving a new baseline quality of life while often never regaining their prior level of functioning.

I consistently attempt to focus on the positive aspects of healthcare delivery and the extraordinary compassion expressed by families and healthcare workers. I pay tribute to my many mentors who have generously shared with me their knowledge and skills in the management of critically ill patients. I honor them by sharing what I have learned with the next generation of healthcare providers.

That night, sleep onset for me did not come as quickly as usual. At 4:00 A.M., when my cell phone rang, I assumed the inevitable. The intern informed me that Mr. Aronson died peacefully while his family held vigil at his bedside. I thanked the intern for the conscientious care she had provided. My sleep during the following hours was intermittent and restless. I awoke spontaneously before the alarm and got out of bed ready to face another day of challenges at the hospital while a family grieved the loss of a loved one.

Another funeral procession of cars with headlights on would journey through the streets of Philadelphia, while onlookers wondered, as Mr. Aronson traveled to his final resting place.

13

Breathing for Two

It was a frigid day in January when Jing arrived in Philadelphia. She had never ventured more than thirty miles from her rural home in China. Now thirty-two years old and thirty-four weeks pregnant, widowed, with both parents deceased, she knew she needed help. When her uncle and aunt offered her a room in their suburban Philadelphia home, she could not refuse.

Although terrified about starting life in a new land where she barely spoke the language, Jing was excited at the prospect of experiencing American city life and having assistance in raising her first child. She adjusted quickly to her new life, made many friends, and adored her uncle and aunt, who never had children of their own. While visiting her obstetrician during her thirty-sixth week of gestation, she noted diffuse aches, sore throat, and a fever. A rapid flu test was positive, and she was started on an antiviral medication known as Tamiflu. Jing had arrived in a major American city during the peak of the influenza season. Her obstetrician instructed her to call if she felt worse.

Although for 99 percent of those infected with influenza, the course is rather benign and self-limited, a very small minority of patients may become deathly ill. Pregnancy renders a mother mildly immunocompromised with a slightly diminished ability to fight viral infections. Unfortunately for Jing, her condition worsened. Over the next forty-eight hours, she became increasingly short of breath and developed fevers to 104 degrees.

Her uncle and aunt drove her to the hospital. The emergency department physician who evaluated Jing knew immediately that something was very wrong. A pulse oximeter monitor placed on Jing's index finger revealed that her oxygen saturation level was markedly reduced at 82 percent. Pulse oximetry is a noninvasive way of assessing oxygen levels in patients who are having respiratory difficulties. When I began medical school in 1978, oxygen assessment was performed by inserting a needle into an artery in the wrist and drawing a blood sample. This painful procedure only assessed the oxygen level for a moment in time. With the advent of pulse oximetry, a noninvasive painless test assesses oxygen levels continuously and helps detect clinical deterioration early leading to quick lifesaving interventions.

A nurse placed nasal prongs in Jing's nose to deliver oxygen supplementation at a gentle flow rate. Immediately, Jing's oxygen level increased to normal at 95 percent. This indicated that 95 percent of Jing's hemoglobin molecules were carrying oxygen. Adequate oxygen delivery was essential not only for her well-being but also for the developing baby she was carrying.

It was reassuring that Jing required minimal oxygen supplementation to provide adequate oxygenation, but it was most concerning that she was breathing rather rapidly at thirty times per minute. With a third-trimester uterus pushing on her hemidiaphragms, it was more difficult for Jing to breathe. Additionally, a chest X-ray obtained revealed evidence of a diffuse, bilateral pneumonia caused by the influenza virus. Because of Jing's tenuous status, need for oxygen, and rapid breathing rate, she was admitted to the obstetrical unit for close monitoring. We hoped that with oxygen supplementation and antiviral therapy, her condition would improve. Neither Jing nor I had any idea that our lives would be forever connected because of the events that would unfold over the next several hours.

Advances in monitoring and care also extended to patient floors outside critical care units. With the development of the rapid response team, nurses could alert a dedicated team of physicians, nurses, and respiratory therapists to respond quickly to life-threatening alterations in vital signs such as heart rate, blood pressure, respiratory rate, and oxygen saturation levels. Additionally, concerning symptoms such as chest pain, shortness of breath, or lethargy could be evaluated more quickly, allowing for an intervention prior to a cardiopulmonary arrest. Undoubtedly, the use of rapid response teams throughout the United States has led to a marked decrease in cardiopulmonary arrests on hospital floors.

More recently, and with the use of modern technology, early warning systems have developed to alert clinicians to a potentially dangerous clinical situation prior to obvious clinical deterioration. As nurses enter vital signs into electronic medical records, algorithms have been developed to send alerts to a physician's cell phone if a combination of abnormal vital signs and lab tests raises a concern for an impending potentially life-threatening disease process such as sepsis.

It was Sunday morning and my weekend to cover the intensive care unit. My drive to work at 7:30 that morning was a breeze. Although weekday commuting was often a challenge, Sunday morning traffic was consistently negligible. Fortunately, I was starting the day feeling refreshed as Saturday night calls were few and sleep disruption was minimal.

As physicians caring for critically ill patients, we expected to receive calls in the middle of the night. The number of calls would vary greatly leading to highly variable amounts of sleep deprivation. Although one might be concerned that a night of diminished sleep would impact on clinical judgment the following day, adaptive responses, including catecholamine (stress response) release and supplementation with caffeine, were always helpful in critical moments.

I was fortunate to work with excellent interns and residents who were the front line in the intensive care unit during the night while I slept. They knew I was just a phone call away if the need for consultation arose. Decades earlier, I had been a medical intern and had also endured the long shifts and sleepless nights that still play an integral role in medical training. Now, more than thirty years later, I had the luxury of relying on younger physicians in training to be my eyes and ears while I was home sleeping, allowing my brain to repair and recharge in anticipation of the following day's work.

Although the anticipation of being called in for an emergency could easily lead to a heightened state of alertness and insomnia, I had grown accustomed to compartmentalizing. I was able to fall asleep easily on call nights and quickly arise to a state of full alertness if my phone disrupted my slumber. My wife of almost forty years has shared a bed through all my nights on call from home and has acquired the knowledge of a physician by osmosis. Despite her sleep disruption from many, many calls through the years, she never complained once. She always understood the importance of the calls I got in the middle of the night.

I arrived at the hospital with a feeling of excitement, not knowing what challenges would present on that day. Although I had received a sign-out of patients by my four pulmonary/critical care colleagues, who were recharging for the weekend, there was considerable uncertainty as to what clinical situations I would be called upon to evaluate.

As a pulmonary/critical care medicine physician in the hospital, I was the most senior and most experienced clinician and expected to deal with a variety of potentially life-threatening problems on very short notice. After decades of experience, I generally felt quite calm. I typically felt, and tried to show, an air of confidence but never arrogance. I interacted with patients, physicians, nurses, respiratory therapists, and other support staff with kindness and respect. The escort staff members had become my buddies and we were on a first-name basis. We often chatted about sports, and they were comfortable asking me for medical advice. I always enjoyed sharing my medical knowledge with anyone comfortable enough to ask.

These interactions frequently took place outside of the traditional doctor-patient relationship: so-called curbside consults. I treasure a box of letters of gratitude from patients and colleagues. Contained in that box is a letter from a woman who had regularly cleaned my office. I suspect she saw my diplomas on the wall and one day expressed concern about her daughter's respiratory difficulties. After our discussion, I suggested that her daughter was likely experiencing undiagnosed asthma.

Weeks later, I found a thank-you note on my desk. She indicated that her daughter was doing great on an asthma inhaler. She thanked me for giving without an expectation of reciprocity. That special moment reminded me of the great joy of agape: a gift of kindness with no anticipation of reward. A human connection with no ulterior motive. A human bond with completely shared interest.

Although I had not considered it at the time, I wished for the same gift of love from a stranger to my children. From time to time, I look at the gratitude notes. These letters constantly reaffirm my decision to become a physician and always bring to the surface the great joy from those transcendent human interactions.

———————

Morning rounds that Sunday in the intensive care unit were uneventful. The ICU team consisted of two first-year interns, two second-year medical residents, nurses, and respiratory therapists, all rounding with me to discuss the events of the past twenty-four hours and plans for each patient. One of the interns and one of the residents had been awake all night. Another intern and resident were starting their shift.

This was the traditional handoff to ensure a smooth transition of care. Information regarding patients' symptoms, exams, laboratory testing, chest X-rays was reviewed. We determined that two patients were stable for transfer to a medical floor. The others required continued monitoring and care in the intensive care unit. The decision to transfer patients to a lower level of monitoring was based on clinical improvement and clinical judgment.

The ultimate decision for disposition/transfer that day rested with me. However, I always sought the opinions of team members as I wanted each member to feel highly valued in the process. Additionally, the younger members would one day have ultimate decision-making responsibility. This was an opportunity for teaching and learning, an opportunity I valued greatly and one that was essential in the training of tomorrow's healthcare providers, as it once had been to me.

The intensive care unit nurses are among the most highly trained healthcare providers in the hospital and often provide invaluable insights that influence decision making about the transfer of a patient. A nurse might point out concerning events that had transpired only hours earlier. This could lead to a decision to maintain ICU monitoring for another twenty-four hours.

Rounds are a great opportunity to teach. This includes asking younger physicians questions about case management in a nonthreatening manner. This is the traditional method handed down for generations. Textbooks and journal articles are definitely of benefit, but it is through a sharing of knowledge and experience at the bedside that most clinicians are shaped.

It is important to be sensitive and never to embarrass a younger healthcare provider. If a question I posed goes unanswered, I quickly give hints or answer the question myself. I pride myself on developing effective methods that included mnemonics and diagrams. Rounds deal with serious issues regarding patients with critical illness but learning in the intensive care unit could still be most rewarding.

After three hours of rounding with the team in the ICU, I headed to the cafeteria for a quick lunch. Although brief, it was enjoyable to interact with the servers and cashiers in the cafeteria. They are my colleagues, many of them have been my friends for years, and they, along with the entire support staff, are absolutely essential to the care we provide to patients and their families.

During basketball season, I would ask one of the environmental workers which team he thought would win the national championship. One spring, he told me Duke was his pick. Though I was not up to date on the teams, I agreed with his choice. When I walked down the hall and saw another server who asked me who I liked in the national championship, without pausing, I said, "Definitely Duke." He nodded and said he certainly agreed.

As I sat finishing my lunch, my cell phone rang. It was one of the senior medical residents consulting on a patient outside the intensive care unit. She was called upon to evaluate a pregnant patient named Jing who had been admitted with influenza.

While speaking with the resident, I quickly flashed back to July 1987. My first weekend of call in the intensive care unit, just out of fellowship, I cared for a young woman who had recently delivered a healthy baby and then developed chicken pox. Because of suppressed immunity associated with pregnancy, chicken pox disseminated throughout her body and she developed respiratory failure because of diffuse lung involvement. She required placement of a breathing tube for attachment to a ventilator. After weeks of critical illness and near death, the lung injury resolved, and she was liberated from mechanical ventilation and soon thereafter walked out of the hospital to be reunited with her young healthy infant.

Now decades later, I wondered if a similar situation had arisen with Jing. Now older, more experienced, and with new medical developments at my fingertips, I listened to the medical resident and jotted down a few notes. From the resident's report, it was evident that this young pregnant woman from China was suffering from life-threatening progressive influenza pneumonia.

Unlike the patient with disseminated chicken pox in 1987, who already had delivered her baby, Jing was still pregnant. She was breathing for two. Medical decisions had to consider the health of the young mother and the health of her baby in utero. Collaboration was essential. I rushed out of the cafeteria and waved to Ruby, the cashier, and Phil, the server. They knew, based upon my fast-paced walking and serious demeanor, that this was not the time for small talk.

As I headed to the stairs, I was ultra-focused on this young pregnant patient. I arrived at Labor and Delivery within minutes. Upon my arrival, a swarm of providers was congregating outside Jing's room.

As I entered the room, I saw a young woman who appeared to be in obvious respiratory distress. She was breathing rapidly, sweating profusely, and using accessory muscles in her neck to assist her fatiguing diaphragm with every breath. I believe my gray hair and advanced age brought some reassurance to Jing and her uncle and aunt. They were pleased that an experienced physician had arrived quickly on a Sunday morning to guide the team at the most terrifying moment of their lives.

Never in medicine was the phrase "A picture is worth a thousand words" more applicable. It was clear that without an intervention, this young mother and her baby could die within minutes. Though the patient's uncle and aunt had never met me before, they entrusted me with their most precious asset: the life of a loved one.

I held Jing's hand and explained that we would need to place a breathing tube in her airway to assist her breathing. At that moment in time, there was a deep connection between Jing and me, two people who spoke different languages and grew up in different countries. I wanted for her exactly what she wanted for herself, to maintain life, for herself and for her baby.

It was evident that Jing would require ventilatory support to deliver oxygen to her vital organs and to those of her baby until her lungs healed. As I was explaining our plans, Jing's respiratory rate proceeded to climb, and her pulse oximetry reading continued to drop. Every breath was a struggle and, although youth was on her side, her breathing muscles had run a marathon and would soon cease to function without ventilatory assistance. Further delay would surely lead to a cardiopulmonary arrest and likely cause permanent disability or death for mother and baby.

I instructed the team to call anesthesia STAT. The overhead page signaled a medical crisis requiring immediate response from the team who would stabilize Jing's airway so we could connect her to a ventilator. Within minutes, the anesthesiologist arrived. After lightly sedating Jing so she would not have to endure the trauma of having a tube placed in her windpipe, my colleague easily passed the breathing tube. We quickly connected Jing to a mechanical ventilator to breathe for her in a rhythmic pattern to ensure adequate delivery of oxygen and excretion of carbon dioxide.

The obstetrical team assisted at the bedside by monitoring Jing's baby in utero. Following initiation of mechanical ventilation, Jing's oxygen levels improved. However, a chest

X-ray obtained following placement of the breathing tube revealed that her influenza pneumonia had rapidly progressed to acute respiratory distress syndrome, ARDS. Although advances in treatment of this life-threatening condition had lowered mortality in recent years, the risk of death was still quite high. We hoped that with adjustments in the ventilator we could provide adequate oxygenation to Jing and her baby as her lungs recovered from this catastrophic viral injury.

Not only did we need to achieve adequate oxygenation and excretion of carbon dioxide, but at the same time we also had to avoid causing oxygen toxicity from high levels of oxygen concentration. The air we breathe is a mixture of gases consisting of 20.9 percent oxygen and 79 percent nitrogen, an inert gas, as well as trace amounts of carbon dioxide, argon, and neon. To maintain life, we must provide adequate oxygen delivery. However, prolonged exposure to high levels of oxygen concentration can cause considerable harm to the lungs and contribute to death. Without adequate delivery of oxygen, the brain will cease to function within minutes.

Moreover, for Jing, it was not just a matter of delivering enough oxygen to her cells, but also delivering enough oxygen to her placenta which nourished her developing baby and avoiding toxicity for both.

Suddenly, Jing's monitor alarm was blaring as her oxygen level was again dropping. The tone of the alarm changed and evoked a visceral response in those in the room. That specific tone could only mean that death was imminent if an intervention did not quickly follow. Although I remained calm, the weight of the situation felt like a ton of bricks. Even as I was trained to compartmentalize and be laser-focused on the crisis at hand, I thought of my beautiful twin daughters who now are mothers and the fact that pregnancy remains the most vulnerable time in a young woman's life. I knew that despite major advances in medical care, young females still die at the time of childbirth.

The obstetrician turned to me and indicated that the baby was showing signs of distress. A decision had to be made; not only were medical decisions to be made but ethical considerations arose as well. Whose life took precedence? Would interventions on the mother's behalf have a negative impact on the baby? Would interventions for the baby have a negative impact on the mother?

Of course, there was no time to convene an ethics panel. The clock was ticking, and lives were at stake. Jing was heavily sedated, and in a few minutes, her baby boy was delivered by an emergency C-section. After the cord was cut, the baby was wrapped in a blanket. To this day, the image of the nurse running to the neonatal intensive care unit with the cloaked newborn firmly grasped in her arms evokes great emotion within me.

Now, we were breathing for just one. As I looked at Jing's oxygen monitor, I noticed further drops in oxygen saturation. The changing alarm tone once again evoked that visceral feeling of nausea and anxiety. Although I no longer had to worry about the baby's survival, I was concerned that without further intervention, Jing would die.

A STAT portable chest X-ray was performed at the bedside to reassess Jing's lungs as well as the position of her breathing tube. We wanted to make sure that she had not developed a collapsed lung that could be easily remedied with a chest tube. It was essential to determine quickly why her oxygen level was dropping and why she was requiring dangerously high levels of potentially toxic oxygen.

What insights would review of her chest X-ray bring? Even with evolving new techniques in imaging, such as CT scan, PET scan, and MRI, a simple chest X-ray could provide valuable information to the bedside within minutes. We gathered around the computer screen to review the chest X-ray. The breathing tube was well positioned and there was no collapsed lung.

Unfortunately, we saw a "whiteout" of both lungs. Air density on a chest X-ray, normally black, on Jing's film was replaced by white: all her tiny air sacs were filled with fluid and inflammatory cells. This new mom was drowning. Influenza had spread throughout both lungs. Her rapid deterioration was consistent with the development of acute respiratory distress syndrome.

We started a medication called Flolan (epoprostenol), a pulmonary vasodilator that can sometimes improve oxygenation. It did not. We chemically paralyzed her to decrease consumption of oxygen by her muscles with the hope that all available oxygen molecules would be diverted to her vital organs: the brain, heart, and kidneys.

We considered prone positioning as more recent data had suggested that oxygenation could be improved by turning a patient onto the abdomen. However, at that time, this was a relatively new unproven technique to improve oxygenation. We have since learned that proning has saved many patients suffering from acute respiratory distress syndrome during the COVID-19 pandemic as gravity redistributes blood flow to the less diseased alveoli and thus improves oxygenation.

There was only one option left. I reached for my cell phone and found the contact listing under E. Earlier in the year, I had attended a Grand Rounds lecture on ECMO—Extracorporeal Membrane Oxygenation. Every Tuesday at noon, doctors convene in the Zubrow Auditorium at Pennsylvania Hospital to learn from experts and stay up to date on important topics. This weekly gathering was for the sole purpose of learning so that we might help our patients and teach others to do the same. At the end of the ECMO lecture, the professor gave a contact number. When I had entered it into my cell phone months earlier, I did not anticipate that it would be my last hope to save the life of this young new mother.

We had to decide whether Jing was a suitable candidate to have her lungs bypassed through a machine for oxygenation. Different factors weighed into the decision-making process such as age, comorbidities, and the ability to tolerate a blood thinner continuously as well as the likelihood of surviving this lifesaving intervention performed after multiple unsuccessful measures had been attempted.

As I dialed the number on my phone and waited for a response, I thought about the unconditional love my wife provided for our children and that our daughters now provided for their children. Would this newborn boy enjoy that same love from Jing or would he someday have to tell people that he never knew his mother because she died in childbirth?

When the ECMO physician answered the phone, he asked whether the patient was stable for transfer to our sister hospital where ECMO could be initiated. I quickly said no. The decision to transfer a critically ill patient is not an easy one. Jing was unstable and could die in the ambulance during transport. The ECMO team would need to come to Jing in our hospital.

The ECMO team arrived quickly and placed a large intravenous line in Jing's internal jugular vein so that blood from her body could pass through a membrane to remove carbon dioxide, a waste product of metabolism, while providing adequate oxygen for cellular functioning. Her lungs could now rest and hopefully heal as the ECMO machine took over the function of her lungs. As Jing struggled to maintain her breath, we held ours, hoping (and, in truth, praying) that this last-ditch option would work.

It did.

After she was stable, Jing was soon placed in an ambulance and transported to our sister hospital for further care. Her newborn baby was cared for in our neonatal unit. Although premature, the baby was doing quite well without a need for his own mechanical ventilator.

Our team had done the best we could. We felt content with the process though we could not determine the final outcome. I have come to learn that focusing on outcomes is emotionally dangerous in a field where death is not uncommon. As Jing and her baby were now in the hands of other providers, we turned our attention to the care of other patients.

But it certainly was difficult not to dwell on the events that had transpired. We received regular updates from our colleagues in the neonatal unit about the baby and from our colleagues in the ECMO Unit about Jing. As evening approached and the sun began to set, we finished our shift in the ICU. Thoughts of the dramatic events of the day had remained front and center. Would Jing and the baby both survive? If they survived, would it be with significant disability? Would Jing develop post-traumatic stress disorder from critical illness? Did we do everything possible to give them both the best chance for recovery?

These are the questions that often haunt us as healthcare providers. By the end of the day, I was confident that we had, indeed, done our very best and that further outcomes were beyond our control. Doctors are human, but in the back of my mind these questions remained.

On a sunny, warm spring day, I crossed paths with the obstetrician who had delivered Jing's baby. I paused for a moment, then blurted out the obvious question: "Do you remember that young woman we cared for together?" I looked directly into his kind smiling eyes and declared, "Tell me what happened to Jing and her baby." He paused. A feeling of joy overcame me. His face could not disguise the obvious. He reached for my hand. Jing and her baby boy were both home and well.

At that moment, I knew that all my years of study and training, all my years of practice, all my sleepless nights in the hospital caring for critically ill patients, had prepared me for that transcendent and highly spiritual moment when my life intersected with Jing's. Though I knew I would probably never see Jing or her son again, they had both become part of my heart and soul, indelibly imprinted in my memory bank, a bank filled with many miraculous, life-altering occurrences along with, like all healthcare professionals, moments of heartbreak.

Perhaps one day Jing would learn the details of that day when, while in a medically induced coma, a dedicated team made timely decisions to care for her and her baby. I assume Jing and her son most likely will never know the specific details of their interventions. Nor will they ever know those who attended to their needs on that special day. However, it is my secret hope that one day before I leave this earth, we will meet and share the joy of this brief but miraculous intersection of our lives.

14

Luckiest Man

The famous baseball player, Lou Gehrig, opened the nation's eyes to the neurodegenerative disease, ALS, also known as Lou Gehrig's disease. After six days of testing at the Mayo Clinic, and on his thirty-sixth birthday, June 19, 1939, Mr. Gehrig was diagnosed with ALS. Despite awareness of his fate, on July 4, 1939, before a packed Yankee Stadium, Mr. Gehrig proclaimed that he considered himself the luckiest man on earth. One might reasonably ask why a man dying of a progressive incurable degenerative disease would consider himself so fortunate.

He had a disease that would rapidly progress unabated and bring an end to his days as a baseball player. Perhaps, in the moment, he was able to focus on the positive aspects of his life and express gratitude. Perhaps he saw his life in the context of his loving parents, his siblings, and his wife. Perhaps he realized what a gift his career was, and he had many cherished friends and fans who adored him. Human reactions to a poor prognosis vary greatly. Lou Gehrig's positive outlook in the face of this devastating illness was inspirational. He died two years following this famous, emotional speech.

When I initially evaluated Jim, an ALS patient, he was having trouble breathing. This incurable muscle disease had already robbed him of his ability to walk. As he entered my office in his motorized wheelchair, he was flanked by his wife, Amy, and his daughter, Julie. Jim was a retired chemist who had worked for a major pharmaceutical company. Until his

ALS, he and Amy had lived quite comfortably in their suburban home just outside Philadelphia.

With today's easy access to information on the Internet, Jim and Amy were very knowledgeable about this progressive disease process that, for most, ended life within three to five years. Like the famous physicist, Stephen Hawking, who had lived with the disease for more than fifty years, they were hopeful of beating the odds. Unlike Mr. Hawking, an atheist, Jim and Amy were strong believers in a Supreme Being who would guide them on this difficult path that lay ahead.

As his muscle weakness progressed, Jim found breathing to be a challenge as well. Jim's shortness of breath increased while he lay in the supine position due to the loss of gravitational assistance to the hemidiaphragms evident when he was upright. This made sleeping quite uncomfortable even with extra pillows. Initiating a nocturnal noninvasive ventilator led to deeper and more refreshing sleep as the efforts of his weakened hemidiaphragms were augmented by this respiratory assist device.

As months passed and muscle weakness progressed, Jim's speech became unintelligible. Through an electronic device, while typing on a special keyboard, his words were magically transformed into computer-generated speech. As Jim's swallowing became impaired, we discussed the placement of a feeding tube that would be advanced through a small hole in the skin overlying his stomach. This would allow Jim to maintain nutrition while avoiding choking on his food.

Jim's sophisticated mechanism of swallowing, involving the coordinated efforts of multiple muscles to allow food to enter the esophagus while bypassing the windpipe, had become greatly impaired. We discussed simultaneous tracheostomy to allow placement of a permanent breathing tube in his windpipe. This would allow for connection to a portable ventilator attached to the back of his motorized wheelchair. An added benefit of tracheostomy included instant access to his airways with a suction device to relieve him of excessive respiratory secretions that he could no longer cough up on his own.

However, most patients with ALS choose to avoid tracheostomy for continuous mechanical ventilation, knowing that, as weakness progresses to total paralysis, life can only be sustained artificially by a mechanical breathing device. Jim had to decide between end-of-life hospice comfort care while dying of respiratory failure related to paralyzed muscles of breathing, or sustained life in a locked-in state eventually limited to eye movements and blinks as his primary connection with those he loved. Life without a tracheostomy and mechanical ventilation would soon end for Jim. Life with a tracheostomy and ventilator support could be sustained possibly for years.

After careful discussions with his wife and daughter and while strongly weighing the potential burden on loved ones, Jim decided he was not ready to leave this earth. Although he strongly believed he had earned a spot in the afterlife of heaven, Jim was hopeful for more time with Amy, his wife of forty years, his thirty-year-old daughter, Julie, and his four grandchildren.

The placement of the feeding tube, known as a PEG tube (percutaneous endoscopic gastrostomy), and a tracheostomy were performed without difficulty. Jim transitioned easily from his noninvasive ventilation device to his new ventilator attached via a two-foot tube to his tracheostomy. Amy learned to disconnect the ventilator from the trach and advance the suction catheter when Jim's lungs sounded gurgly.

Although it was no longer safe to eat full meals, Jim still enjoyed his preserved sense of taste and limited his oral intake to three teaspoons of pudding several times per day. Liquid nutrition was infused through his new abdominal opening connected to his stomach. Visiting nurses and respiratory therapists stopped by regularly to assist Amy in caring for Jim. His daughter, Julie, stopped by each evening after work. On weekends, his grandchildren would fight over taking turns for the opportunity to sit on Jim's lap to cruise the grounds in the motorized wheelchair, now equipped with two bicycle horns that the kids could enjoy honking.

This quality of life had seemed unimaginable to Jim just six months earlier. Surprisingly, his loss of muscle function and ability to breathe on his own were not his primary daily focus.

As Itzhak Perlman, the great musician impaired by polio, once said, "Focus on ability, not disability." Jim focused on his ability to love and be loved. He could still experience the pleasure of the gentle touch of his loving wife's caress and feel the joy of his grandchildren's laughter. He could appreciate the sounds of wind blowing through trees and the wonderful scents of spring flowers. He could still taste vanilla, chocolate, and strawberry, his favorite flavors. Although the burden on Amy was great, her faith and community of friends gave her strength to persevere.

As Jim's fingers eventually could no longer type to generate speech on his computer, he quickly mastered communication through eye movements and blinks on the screen of his eye gaze device. He had never imagined that, with various permutations of blinking and shutting and rolling his eyes, along with upward, downward, and lateral gazes, he could communicate his wishes, thoughts, and feelings. Even his grandchildren were so patient, as Jim expressed himself in the only way still possible.

Jim spent many waking hours watching sporting events and movies on television with his wife. He enjoyed reading chemistry journals and biographies of famous scientists. He contemplated the limitations of advance directives as his wishes changed with disease progression. Many patients with ALS choose to pursue a less aggressive approach as disease progresses. The thought of being wheelchair bound, unable to move, unable to breathe without a machine, and with muscle activity limited to eye movements for communication is an unacceptable existence to most, but for Jim, the ongoing loving experience with his family made it still worthwhile.

I realize as a physician that goals and priorities in the life of a dying patient may change as disease progresses and that ongoing communication and clarification of a patient's goals and priorities are essential. What a patient expresses as his or her wishes today when talking, breathing, and walking, may be very different in six months when the actual experience of disease progression rather than its anticipation reshapes previously expressed wishes, goals, and priorities.

It was a sunny day in September when Jim's condition suddenly deteriorated. He began to cough and developed shaking chills and fevers. Amy knew immediately by looking at Jim that something was very wrong. EMS arrived within minutes. Jim's blood pressure was low and he appeared stuporous. In the emergency room, he was diagnosed with pulmonary sepsis. A chest X-ray demonstrated evidence of bilateral pneumonia, affecting both of Jim's lungs. Bacteria in his lungs had multiplied logarithmically and invaded his bloodstream. The microbial pathogens disseminated to his organs and led to major derangements in heart and kidney function.

Despite administration of intravenous fluids and broad-spectrum antibiotics in a timely manner, it was clear that Jim was dying. Even after three potent medicines were given simultaneously to support a feebly functioning heart, his blood pressure continued to drop. His kidneys were failing and unable to sustain life without immediate initiation of dialysis.

As I entered Jim's ICU room, I paused for a few minutes and watched as Amy sat by his side looking at the man that she had loved for so many years. Soon after I made eye contact with Jim, with a sequence of eye movements and blinks he expressed a clear understanding and chose to avoid initiation of dialysis. With the progressive decline in blood pressure, an increase in heart rate, mottled discoloration of his arms and legs, and bluish discoloration of his fingertips and toes, it was clear that Jim would die soon of multisystem organ failure brought about by septic shock from pneumonia.

Jim had hoped for the good fortune of Stephen Hawking who lived more than fifty years with ALS. That was not to be. Amy would not leave Jim's bedside. She drank multiple cups of coffee for fear that the love of her life would leave this earth while she slept. It was 3:00 A.M. on a Sunday morning with the ICU dark and quiet and Jim knew that death was imminent. As Amy rubbed his shoulder, he blinked to communicate his last earthly feelings to his soul mate, "Thank you for caring for me. Thank you for giving up so much. Thank you for loving me. Hugs and kisses to our wonderful daughter and grandchildren. I love you, good-bye, see you on the other side." Before Amy could respond, Jim closed his eyes and was forever gone from this earth.

15

POP!

The pilot had just announced that the cruising altitude of 30,000 feet had been reached when Cindy began to develop left-sided chest pain. This discomfort was like pain she had experienced multiple times before, just prior to menstruation. This time, however, it was much more severe. With each inspiration came the feeling of a dagger poking deeply beneath her left breast. As the pain progressed and she began to sweat, the elderly woman sitting next to her pressed the flight attendant call button.

When asked if she felt okay, wishing to conserve her shallow breaths, Cindy shook her head "No." The flight attendant glanced at Cindy and knew that medical attention was urgently needed. Within seconds, the pilot asked for any physicians on the flight to identify themselves.

Josh, who was finishing his medical residency and flying to Boston to interview for a pulmonary/critical care medicine fellowship, had often wondered whether he would ever be called upon to evaluate a passenger during air flight. He quickly identified himself. Josh was a compassionate soul and was on his way to becoming a superb young physician. Ironically, he had recently attended a Grand Rounds lecture on medical emergencies during air travel. This recently acquired knowledge would help save Cindy's life.

Josh turned to the flight attendant and asked him to locate the plane's medical bag. He again identified himself as a physician to Cindy and obtained her permission to proceed with an evaluation. When flying, Cindy always chose the aisle seat as she had learned that this location facilitated leg stretching and lowered the risk of blood clots. Josh knelt beside her and with a soft, soothing voice began to obtain a medical history.

Cindy revealed how she was experiencing excruciating left-sided chest pain, worse with each inspiration, like prior episodes just before her periods. She denied a history of blood clots in her legs and lungs, noted no history of cardiac disease, and indicated that she was a healthy twenty-eight-year-old without medical problems and on no medications, including oral contraceptive therapy.

Josh felt her radial pulse and observed it to be strong but rapid. Her skin was cold and clammy. A pulmonary embolism, a blood clot in the lung, was a consideration, but Josh knew that such an event associated with air flight was usually days to weeks after and not during the flight.

When he listened with the stethoscope handed to him by the flight attendant, the diagnosis became evident. With total absence of breath sounds over the left lung, it was almost a certainty that Cindy was experiencing a pneumothorax or collapsed lung. While studying for his board exam, Josh had read about a rare condition known as catamenial pneumothorax or collapsed lung associated with the menstrual cycle. Without hesitation, Josh turned to the flight attendant and requested that he place Cindy on nasal oxygen and instruct the pilot to return immediately to the airport. Within seconds came the announcement: "This is Captain Anderson, your pilot. We will be returning to the Philadelphia International Airport due to a medical emergency."

Josh held Cindy's hand as he explained that she likely suffered from thoracic endometriosis syndrome. During her menstrual cycles, rising levels of the hormones progesterone and estrogen stimulate growth of the endometrial tissue lining her uterus. In the absence of an implanted fertilized egg, the tissue sloughs during menstruation and blood flows through the cervix.

Abnormal endometrial tissue outside the uterus is known as endometriosis. Abnormal endometrial tissue on the surface of the lungs causes thoracic endometriosis syndrome. Josh postulated that the chest pain associated with prior periods was due to progesterone and estrogen stimulation of endometrial tissue on the surface of her lungs; this likely caused a small hole that transiently leaked air but subsequently healed like a cut on the skin.

Boyle's Law, named for a physicist, describes the relationship between pressure and volume changes and applies to the lungs during air flight. As the plane ascends to 30,000 feet, the barometric pressure decreases, and the volume of the lungs increases. Like a balloon, as the lung volume increases it may pop. Most likely, Cindy's left lung had recently popped just before her period due to hormonal stimulation of ectopic endometrial tissue on its surface (ectopic meaning normal tissue, but where such tissue should not be found).

The freshly healed miniscule hole in Cindy's lung was unable to tolerate lung expansion as the barometric pressure dropped during ascent of the airplane. While in air flight, ongoing leaking of air through the hole in her lung could lead to a buildup of pressure in her chest. This could compromise function of her heart and lead to a cardiac arrest. Josh was very much aware that Cindy required placement of a tube into her chest to release the buildup of pressure and reinflate her lung. This required urgent transfer to an emergency room after landing. Within thirty minutes, the plane landed and returned to the terminal. An ambulance was waiting and as they departed the airport, Josh called the emergency room attending physician at the closest hospital.

A portable chest X-ray obtained soon after Cindy's arrival at the hospital confirmed the presence of a complete collapse of the left lung. Within minutes of placement of a chest tube by the emergency room attending, Cindy noted a dramatic decrease in her pain as her lung reinflated. With the knowledge that Cindy would be well cared for, Josh hopped into a cab to return to the airport, hoping to catch the next flight to Boston. He thought to himself that if he were late for his interview, certainly he had a compelling reason.

Cindy was admitted to a medical floor for further evaluation and care. Her chest tube, connected to a suction device mounted on the wall near the head of her bed, was set at negative 20 cm of water pressure to keep her lung inflated. Dr. Morgan, a thoracic surgeon, arrived the following morning to evaluate Cindy, and she concurred with Josh's assessment. Dr.

Morgan expressed surprise that a third-year medical resident had been astute enough to diagnose such a rare condition.

The following day, Cindy underwent video-assisted thoracoscopic surgery in the operating room. Dr. Morgan was able to visualize the surface of the lung by inserting a camera through a small incision in the chest. She biopsied multiple nodular densities on the surface of Cindy's lung, oversewed the small hole that was the source of the lung collapse, and instilled a sclerosing agent so the surface of the lung would adhere to the inner lining of the chest wall, thereby preventing a future lung collapse. Review of the biopsies, indeed, revealed that pieces of tissue had migrated from her endometrium and were covering the surface of her lung. Cindy was discharged home the next day with plans to visit a gynecologist to discuss hormonal treatment of her rare condition, thoracic endometriosis syndrome. Josh moved to Boston the next year for his pulmonary/critical care medicine fellowship and never saw Cindy again.

Subsequently, Cindy became my patient. She had sought pulmonary follow-up for her rare condition that almost took her life during air flight. Now, as ten years have passed, Cindy continues to do well with no recurrence of lung collapse. On out-of-town trips to visit family and friends, she travels by car.

16

Broken Heart

It was 6:58 A.M. on a cold winter Saturday morning. I woke up spontaneously, looked at the clock, and realized I had slept through the night without my beeper blasting. Still in bed, I could see that my wife was still sound asleep. As I watched her gentle breathing, I reflected on her selflessness as she had endured many sleepless nights tending to our young children or listening to me talking on the telephone to ICU interns and residents. It had been a restful night for both of us.

I quietly left the bedroom, showered and dressed, ate breakfast, and drove to the hospital for ICU rounds. Upon my arrival, a quick walk through the intensive care unit revealed many empty beds. The ICU census was unpredictable and could change in a heartbeat. I met with the team of residents and interns and was informed that we had only three patients to discuss. This was a welcome break from the often-frenetic pace of our busy intensive care unit. It allowed for extra teaching time and a realistic chance of spending the afternoon with my wife and children.

Soon after we finished discussing management of the first patient, the overhead speakers blared: CRT 6 Core, CRT 6 Core. The Cardiac Resuscitation Team was being urgently summoned. At that moment, nothing could have been more pressing. My heart began beating faster as a surge of adrenaline diffused through my body. A patient in the building had stopped breathing. We were charged with intervening before permanent cessation of respiratory and cardiac function occurred, resulting in death.

We quickly headed to the stairs. There was no time to wait for the elevator. A delay of seconds could mean the difference between life and death. A delay in a successful resuscitation could contribute to permanent brain injury from decreased supply of oxygen to the brain.

As we arrived on the sixth floor, we were directed to room 623 where other healthcare providers, including respiratory therapists and nurses, were attending to Mr. Davis. Jason, his medical intern, was present and quickly reviewed that the patient who was undergoing CPR had a history of severe congestive heart failure and frequent hospital admissions. Mr. Davis had been admitted the night before with increasing shortness of breath, bilateral leg swelling, and inability to lie flat in bed. A buildup of fluid in his legs and lungs reflected the diminished functioning of a failing heart.

A recent cardiac echo had demonstrated a greatly diminished left ventricular ejection fraction of 15 percent. Normally, with each contraction, the heart expels at least 50 percent of its blood. The decline in Mr. Davis's cardiac function was reflected in the ability of his heart to expel only 15 percent with each contraction. The diuretic Lasix had been administered the night before with resultant urine output of three liters. Minutes earlier, the intern had been alerted by the telemetry staff that remote heart monitoring demonstrated short runs of a potentially fatal arrhythmia, ventricular tachycardia.

When Jason, the intern, arrived, Mr. Davis had noted that his breathing had improved. But soon thereafter, Mr. Davis closed his eyes and stopped breathing. Absence of a palpable carotid pulse led to initiation of CPR, yells for help, and a call to the operator to announce CRT 6 Core.

The senior medical resident who was certified in ACLS (Advanced Cardiac Life Support) led the resuscitation efforts. Established algorithms were utilized to guide the team during resuscitation. Medications such as epinephrine, and electrical shocks based upon the rhythm detected on the heart monitor, continued during the resuscitation efforts. Blood was drawn and was sent STAT to check for abnormalities such as diuretic-induced hypokalemia that may have contributed to Mr. Davis's cardiac arrest.

Despite ongoing efforts to revive Mr. Davis, however, his heart could not be restarted and he was pronounced dead. There are times when even the dramatic advances in medicine and the intensive efforts of a trained CRT team cannot prevent the inevitable.

———————

The decision to stop CPR is a challenging one. It is an acknowledgement of failure and acceptance of an unexpected death. Monitoring of CO_2 exhaled during each breath with an end-tidal CO_2 (ETCO2) monitor can assist the medical team in assessing adequacy of chest compressions and determining the end point of resuscitation efforts.

For CO_2 to be detected with each exhalation, three conditions must be met:

- Cells continue to produce carbon dioxide as a by-product of metabolism.

- Blood continues to flow from the cells to the lungs to deliver carbon dioxide produced for excretion.

- Air continues to move in and out of the patient's lungs.

When a cardiac arrest occurs, end-tidal CO_2 quickly drops to zero. At this moment in time, CO_2 is still being produced at the cellular level but is not returning back to the lungs for excretion because of lack of cardiac pumping. Therefore, as the patient is ventilated, either by mechanical ventilation or through a bag valve mask device, no carbon dioxide is excreted and the digital graph reads a level of zero. In the absence of a palpable carotid pulse, cardiac arrest is confirmed, and CPR is initiated.

With effective chest compressions aiding in blood flow return to the lungs, carbon dioxide is once again excreted, and this will be reflected on the digital monitor. The goal breath rate for the patient during resuscitation is ten per minute or approximately one breath every six seconds. Each breath is delivered slowly over one second with a large enough volume to cause the chest to rise. For a reasonable chance of survival, end-tidal CO_2 during CPR should exceed 15 mmHg (millimeters of mercury). If end-tidal CO_2 is persistently less than 10 mmHg after twenty minutes of good technique CPR, survival is highly unlikely. Note that normal end-tidal CO_2 is 35–45 mmHg.

As we have evolved as a civilization, so has our determination of the moment human life ends. Shakespeare's King Lear invokes lack of breath as the sign of death: "If that her breath will mist or stain the stone, why then she lives." Others in the distant past argued that decapitation, rigor mortis, or putrefaction (decay of the body) were the sure signs of death and most likely to prevent premature burial. After the stethoscope was invented in 1816 by René Laënnec, this simple device, which still to this day is much more than of symbolic value, aided in diagnosing death. After heart sounds were determined to be forever lost, the end of human life was felt to be certain.

However, caution is advised when pronouncing death. The Lazarus syndrome, named for the soul in the New Testament raised from the dead by Jesus, describes patients with delayed return of spontaneous circulation after apparently failed attempts at revival. Based upon the medical literature, there have been rare cases in which patients are declared dead prematurely, after presumed unsuccessful CPR. The prudent physician should wait at least ten minutes after stopping CPR before declaring end of life by absence of cardiac activity.

Additionally, the condition of environmentally induced hypothermia presents another caution. In 2015, a fourteen-year-old boy survived forty-two minutes of full submersion in cold water. As the body is cooled, metabolic demands and oxygen requirement decrease. This observation has led to the adage that a patient with hypothermia cannot be declared dead until warmed to normal body temperature when baseline metabolic requirements return.

Hundreds of thousands of out-of-hospital cardiac arrests occur each year in the United States. Only 10 percent survive for hospital admission. Less than half of these admitted to the hospital will have a good neurological outcome. Established advanced life support algorithms offer standardized guides for physicians in the effort of cardiopulmonary resuscitation.

Following a primary cardiac arrest, if there is a lack of return of spontaneous circulation and a lack of a shockable rhythm after twenty minutes of resuscitation efforts, survival is unlikely. A patient with asystole or flat line for twenty minutes is unlikely to survive. The chance of surviving a primary cardiac arrest is related to how much time has transpired from when the heart stops to when a return of spontaneous circulation becomes evident, and the patient no longer requires CPR to maintain vital organ perfusion (adequate blood flow).

If a return of spontaneous circulation occurs, but the patient remains comatose, therapeutic hypothermia may increase the chances of neurological recovery. Initiation of hypothermia may proceed after obtaining informed consent from a surrogate decision maker. The body is cooled by a protocol to approximately 32–34 degrees centigrade for twenty-four hours and then gradually rewarmed. This intervention is initiated as soon as possible.

The primary goal of therapeutic hypothermia is to prevent permanent neurological injury. When cardiac arrest occurs, blood flow to the brain immediately stops. Oxygen stores are lost within seconds. ATP and glucose needed for cellular functioning are depleted within five minutes and cellular death begins. Therapeutic hypothermia decreases the resultant inflammation and slows metabolic activity and, therefore, diminishes oxygen and ATP requirements. Risks of therapeutic hypothermia include arrhythmias, bleeding, seizures, and metabolic derangements such as hypoglycemia (low blood sugar) and hyperkalemia (elevated potassium level).

After completion of twenty-four hours of hypothermia and the subsequent gradual rewarming of the body, the patient is followed in the intensive care unit on a mechanical ventilator for neurological recovery. Typically, an attending neurology consultant assists the primary medical team and family members in the decision-making process should neurological recovery fail to occur by seven days. Lack of neurological recovery would strongly suggest that a catastrophic anoxic brain injury has occurred (lack of oxygen to the brain). Continuous EEG monitoring may assist the clinicians in ruling out ongoing seizures as the cause of ongoing coma. If it is determined that there is no reasonable hope of neurological recovery, discussions regarding withdrawal of life support typically would follow.

17

Boerhaave Syndrome— Dangerous Retching

The ICU had been quiet all day. Perhaps a bit too quiet. Then, simultaneously around 3:00 P.M., when everyone experiences a dip in circadian rhythm manifesting as mild sluggishness magnified by inactivity, two patients were wheeled in on stretchers. One, a middle-aged man having a heart attack, was quickly transported to the cardiac cath lab. The other, Elaine, an elderly female patient in shock, was evaluated by me as the pulmonary/critical care medicine attending physician along with the ICU residents.

To the layperson, shock is a state of extreme surprise. To the clinician, circulatory shock is a life-threatening disease state characterized by inability to deliver adequate oxygen to major organs and manifests as low blood pressure, rapid heart rate, decreased urine output, and cold and clammy skin. All patients presenting with circulatory shock are at risk for rapid clinical deterioration and death if the cause is not immediately determined.

Four major types of circulatory shock include:

- *Hypovolemic*. This includes patients who have lost significant amounts of bodily fluid through bleeding, diarrhea, sweating, urination, or vomiting.

- *Cardiac*. This includes patients having a massive heart attack, dysfunction of a heart valve, or a poorly contracting heart muscle.

119

- *Obstructive.* This includes patients with massive pulmonary embolism (blood clot), cardiac tamponade (fluid compressing the heart), or tension pneumothorax (collapsed lung) interfering with cardiac function.

- *Distributive.* A state in which systemic vasodilatation (distension of the blood vessels) leads to decreased blood flow to the brain, heart, and kidneys as in the life-threatening infection known as sepsis.

Our primary task was to rapidly resuscitate the patient with intravenous fluids, add medications known as pressors to improve blood pressure, and then determine the etiology of the circulatory shock. Without quickly identifying the cause, an appropriate intervention could not be determined, and death would likely soon follow.

———————

Elaine appeared quite ill. Her lethargy precluded any meaningful conversation. Review of the electronic records revealed that she had undergone colectomy for colon cancer two days earlier. Other than postoperative nausea and vomiting, her clinical course had remained unremarkable until she complained of chest pain just hours before we first met her in the intensive care unit.

Urgent CT scanning revealed no abnormalities in the abdomen or pelvis but did demonstrate a large collection of fluid surrounding and compressing her right lung. Her STAT blood testing revealed a markedly elevated white blood count, strongly suggestive of a severe life-threatening infection. With a presumed diagnosis of septic shock, broad-spectrum antibiotics were administered. Why did this patient have a large collection of fluid compressing her right lung and was it related to her septic shock?

The thirteenth-century philosopher, William of Ockham (also known as William of Occam), is often credited with describing a basic tenet, known as Occam's Razor, which suggests that the simplest explanation is usually correct. This is true in the practice of day-to-day medicine as well, as physicians typically search for a unifying theme that explains all findings.

Boerhaave Syndrome—Dangerous Retching

It was imperative to analyze the fluid compressing Elaine's lung. As this collection of fluid was drained, a foul smell permeated the room. This strongly suggested the presence of infection. Evaluation of the fluid revealed many white blood cells and bacteria as well as a very high amount of the enzyme known as amylase. This digestive enzyme, produced in the salivary glands and pancreas, is involved in carbohydrate digestion. Why was there so much amylase in the fluid and where had it come from?

Elaine was asked to swallow Gastrografin contrast. This opaque liquid administered by radiologists appears bright white on X-rays. As Elaine repeatedly swallowed the fluid, we were able to watch as it descended her esophagus. Our suspicion was confirmed as fluid leaked through a hole in the bottom part of her esophagus. Why did Elaine have a hole in her esophagus that allowed leakage of bacteria and food into her chest to cause this life-threatening infection?

We concluded that while vomiting after surgery, severe retching was the culprit. This well-described process, known as Boerhaave syndrome, though rare, has been reported in the medical literature. The amylase in the fluid collection had been produced in Elaine's salivary glands and swallowed, mixed with bacteria normally residing in her mouth. Anything swallowed normally transits the esophagus into the stomach. The tear in Elaine's esophagus caused by powerful retching after surgery allowed saliva and bacteria to enter directly into her chest cavity, resulting in a collection of infected fluid known as empyema.

Soon thereafter, Dr. Morgan of thoracic surgery arrived to place a chest tube to drain the remaining fluid surrounding Elaine's right lung. After obtaining consent from Elaine's husband, Dr. Morgan performed a thoracotomy to open the chest and close the esophageal hole with sutures. When Elaine returned to the intensive care unit from the operating room eight hours later, an endotracheal tube remained in her windpipe, connected to a ventilator. She was heavily sedated and still requiring medication to maintain normal blood pressure and continued multiple intravenous antibiotics at the direction of the infectious disease consultant. When her urine output decreased postoperatively, it was evident that she had developed an acute kidney injury related to her critical illness. Dialysis of Elaine's kidneys, therefore, was initiated by the consulting nephrologist.

On post-op day three, although Elaine appeared to be improving and her blood pressure was normal off pressor support, she was found sitting in a pool of blood emanating from her rectum. A STAT GI consultation was performed. The challenge was to determine whether the blood was coming from her colon below or had passed from her stomach and esophagus above.

With ongoing bleeding, Elaine required multiple blood transfusions. Because of reluctance to pass an endoscope through the esophagus where surgery had recently taken place, we decided to perform an arteriogram with the hope of identifying the bleeding vessel. Indeed, the GI source of bleeding was identified through arteriography and with subsequent injection of Gelfoam into a small vessel supplying the stomach, the bleeding stopped immediately.

Elaine was returned to the intensive care unit following the procedure and within twenty-four hours was weaned off her ventilator. She continued to require dialysis to substitute for her injured kidneys. The following day, she was sufficiently improved to allow transfer to the intermediate critical care unit for further management. Physical therapists worked with Elaine daily to help her regain strength she had lost while critically ill in the hospital. As her kidney function returned to normal by post-op day ten, she no longer required dialysis. Due to her overall weakness, a social worker arranged for Elaine to be transferred to a rehab center, with ultimate plans for a return to her home once she had regained strength and mobility.

18

Am I Critical?

For many years, I took care of a lovely elderly woman named Agatha, who had advanced COPD. We developed a profound and meaningful human connection. I came to understand her intense anxiety related to her respiratory disease. While checking her blood pressure in the office, Agatha typically would ask me, "Am I critical?"

I would stop pumping the sphygmomanometer (blood pressure monitor), look into her eyes, and smile. I always reassured her that she was not critical. Although chronically ill, she was breathing comfortably at rest and oxygenating well.

I came to understand Agatha's need for reassurance. We developed a deep and lasting bond. She and her family trusted me to guide her through years of illness. As is often the case with COPD, Agatha developed a life-threatening deterioration requiring hospitalization in the intensive care unit. Her decline and respiratory dysfunction were so severe that we had to place a breathing tube in her windpipe so a ventilator could breathe for her.

After seven days of medical therapy and rest of her weary muscles of breathing, we were able to wean her off her mechanical ventilatory support. Her recovery was slow, and eight weeks passed before she returned to her baseline. When she returned to the office a month later, she looked me in the eye and said, "Doc, was I critical?"

Without pausing, I smiled and replied, "A little bit." We both laughed. Though our concepts of the word critical were somewhat different, Agatha and I could share this quiet, personal, somewhat comical moment as we both reflected on her near-death experience.

Agatha's condition deteriorated the following year. We both knew this could happen. As her breathing progressively worsened, we discussed oxygen supplementation and a focus on comfort care. I guided her away from the intensive care unit and toward care in the home with hospice support to live her final days with peace, dignity, and comfort as she was surrounded by loved ones.

Agatha passed away peacefully while receiving oxygen supplementation, liquid morphine, and the sedative Ativan. The week after Agatha died, her daughter, Cynthia, brought me cookies with a thank-you note. She told me that one of Agatha's final requests was for her to bake cookies for me. The note contained words of gratitude from the family. I shared these delicious cookies with my staff and placed the note in my special box where I return from time to time when I need a reminder of my great privilege to be a physician.

19

Too Young to Die

David was shy as a boy, always overshadowed by his older, more athletic brothers. His diminutive stature led to frequent bullying on the playground and seemed to contribute to his lack of self-confidence.

That all changed when David entered high school and went through a growth spurt that allowed him to pass his peers in height. His emerging talent as a left-handed pitcher brought him local fame on the baseball field. By tenth grade, he was six feet, five inches tall, just an inch shy of his tall, slender father. His ninety-mile-per-hour fastball from the mound made batters tremble.

His parents began to realize that an athletic scholarship with a full ride to college was likely. His dad, Peter, a policeman, and his mother, Rebecca, an elementary school teacher, could use a break on tuition. Two of David's brothers were in college. David's high school coach met with his parents and suggested that he may want to skip college and go straight to professional baseball.

A six-figure signing bonus was enticing but a free college education was hard to pass up. David's parents viewed a college education as a top priority, but both agreed the final decision was up to their son. This season opener was against their local rivals. The opposing pitcher was no friend. He had been the local playground bully when David was in grade school. Although the thought of hitting his old rival with a ninety-mile-per hour fastball was a fleeting fantasy, David would never intentionally hurt anyone. Having been bullied as a child had made him sensitive and kind.

Tragically, his kindness did not stop what was about to happen as he stepped up to bat. With a player on first and second base, he planned to bunt, hoping to advance his teammates to second and third base. Then came a fastball heading toward his knees. He tried to evade the path of the ball but could not. As he fell to the ground, hundreds of fans jumped to their feet. His parents screeched in disbelief. The team doctor ran to the field. Ice was applied and soon thereafter an ambulance arrived. David writhed in pain. Fans cringed while replaying in their minds the sound of bone cracking on impact as the baseball shattered David's right femur.

In the local emergency room, an elderly physician told Peter and Rebecca that David had a fracture of the femur of his right leg, but his prognosis was excellent. Even if the leg did not heal perfectly, as a left-hand pitcher, most of the weight would be on his left leg during the windup of each pitch.

That night was a sleepless one for David and his parents. Injections of morphine relieved David's pain. The following day, he was wheeled to the operating room. After a two-hour operation, the attending orthopedic surgeon met with Peter and Rebecca who had been anxiously awaiting an update. The news was quite good. David's fracture would heal completely and after physical therapy and strengthening, he would be back on the mound hurling his ninety-mile-per-hour fastball.

David was in a post-anesthesia fog when he arrived in the recovery room. After asking for multiple doses of IV Dilaudid, he was placed on a PCA (Patient Controlled Analgesia) pump that allowed David to get immediate pain relief with the push of a button. When he was placed on the device, the dosing was adjusted in order to account for David's naïve narcotic status. Because he had never received narcotics, the impact of these potent analgesics could be considerable. An overdose could lead to suppression of respiratory drive to breathe and respiratory arrest.

The development of potent narcotics was a godsend for pain sufferers. Trauma, postoperative, and cancer-related pain all respond well to potent synthetic narcotics such as morphine and Dilaudid. Narcotics relieve pain by attaching to mu receptors. These same receptors are found abundantly in the medulla, the brain's center for control of breathing. Excessive and frequent doses of these potent narcotics may be quite dangerous as we seek to relieve suffering without causing harm. This requires careful dosing and careful monitoring of pain relief and respirations.

David was admitted to a postoperative floor and placed on continuous pulse oximetry, allowing nurses to monitor his oxygen levels while assessing his mental status. Life-threatening respiratory depression leading to respiratory arrest is preceded by lethargy and coma. The nurses knew that if David could be easily aroused to full consciousness, he was unlikely to develop respiratory depression leading to a respiratory arrest.

Unfortunately, this meant that a nurse had to awaken David hourly for adequate neurological assessment. One cannot distinguish between sleep and coma without waking the patient to full consciousness. The nurses apologized to David as they disrupted his sleep hourly for assessment. 6:00 A.M. came quickly and so did the rounding surgeon and residents. The youthful-appearing trainees in scrubs joked with David about his notorious fastball. One resident asked David if he would be the next Sandy Koufax or Randy Johnson. By noon, David's discharge papers were signed. He was sent home with a follow-up appointment and a prescription for the oral narcotic oxycodone.

David returned to the ball field to a standing ovation the following week. He sat in the dugout with his teammates as he watched his team lose a close game. He had adapted easily to crutches. After the game, all his teammates signed his cast and wished him a speedy recovery.

Nighttime was a challenge for David. Shifting in bed with his thigh-high cast caused pain. David took his oxycodone more frequently than prescribed. At his follow-up appointment one week post-op, he asked the nurse practitioner for another prescription. She cautioned him about opioid addiction, but David convinced her that the pain at times was unbearable. He was provided with instructions to take no more than one oxycodone every six hours for the next week.

Three days later, David found his oxycodone bottle empty. He had taken his opioids more frequently than prescribed. He felt panic as a craving came over him as never before. He called the nurse practitioner and pleaded for another refill. She politely but firmly said, "No." She suggested extra-strength Tylenol. Always a polite boy, now David screamed at the nurse practitioner using expletives. He became more anxious and easily agitated. His parents were concerned. They had never seen David act in such an aggressive manner.

David's parents called the nurse practitioner and asked to speak to David's surgeon. Dr. Hardy agreed with the nurse practitioner and said that, by now, David should not need a narcotic for pain control. He, too, recommended extra-strength Tylenol and physical therapy. That night, David called a teammate to take him for a ride. Clifford, a second baseman, was headed neither for college nor major league baseball. David knew Clifford hung out with a local gang.

David asked Clifford how he could obtain narcotics on the street. Clifford told David to meet a friend outside a local bar at midnight. David paid $10 a pill for thirty oxycodone. His savings took a big hit but he felt that he had no choice. Thirty pills went by quickly. David called Clifford for a favor. He wanted thirty more oxycodone but was short on cash. Clifford said he had an idea. David's shot at major league baseball was known throughout the community. Clifford introduced David to a middle-aged man who flashed a thick wallet. The man pulled out a wad of $100 bills and gave $10,000 in exchange for 50 percent of David's major league signing bonus. David had to agree to forego college and accept any major league offer.

David asked the man where to sign. The man smiled and said, "no contract. It will be our secret agreement." David was thrilled. With $10,000 he could buy 1,000 oxycodone. Clifford arranged for the transaction, which took place the following night. In the following days, David's parents became concerned. David was cutting classes. His parents were worried that David was becoming depressed about missing his baseball season. They assured him his leg would heal and he would be fine. With each passing day, David became increasingly distraught and frequently agitated.

Sunday morning church service always had been important for David and his parents. When David did not join them for breakfast, his father knocked on his bedroom door. When there was no answer, David's father Peter entered to find him unresponsive. Peter, a police officer, had been a medic in the Army in Iraq. He quickly realized that David was not breathing and had no pulse.

After many months in Iraq on the frontlines, Peter had learned to stay calm in a moment of crisis. As he began CPR, he yelled to his wife to call 911. David's mother bolted up the stairs into the bedroom. She screamed when she saw her husband aggressively and rhythmically compressing David's chest. EMS arrived within five minutes and resumed CPR, placed an intravenous line, and injected several doses of epinephrine and Narcan.

Within minutes, David had a return of spontaneous circulation. His heart was beating once again, his blood pressure was good, but David remained unresponsive. A breathing tube was placed in David's windpipe so air could be squeezed into his lungs through a rubber device known as an Ambu Bag.

David was carried on a stretcher to the ambulance waiting in front of the house. As he was loaded into the vehicle, his parents jumped into their car to follow the ambulance as it sped into town with lights on and siren blasting. Sadly, an unresponsive teenager was not an uncommon sight for the emergency room staff; it was all-too-familiar during the opioid epidemic.

The emergency room doctor was coincidentally the same physician who had cared for David's fractured leg. Rebecca asked if her son would be okay. Dr. Gilbert replied that David's heart was strong and there was no evidence of cardiac injury. His blood work showed good kidney function. Dr. Gilbert suspected that David had taken too many pain pills. She told David's parents that he would be transported to the intensive care unit and would remain on the ventilator for close monitoring of his vital signs and level of consciousness.

The respiratory therapist connected David's breathing tube to a ventilator that would breathe for him until he could breathe on his own. David was placed on a ventilator mode that would deliver a breath of oxygen every five seconds. If David's brain sent a message to breathe more quickly, the machine would recognize and assist the effort to deliver additional breaths.

However, even if David's brain sent no message to breathe, he was assured of getting a breath every five seconds or twelve times per minute. Each delivered breath would inflate David's lungs; and after breath delivery, David would exhale from the elastic recoil like a deflating balloon so carbon dioxide could be released.

Early that afternoon, the intensive care unit attending physician entered David's room. His parents were anxiously awaiting an update of David's condition. Dr. Franklin was an elderly physician who had cared for critically ill patients over a forty-year career. After examining David, he turned to Peter and Rebecca and explained that vital organs such as the heart and kidneys were functioning well, but that a urine drug screen had come back positive for narcotics.

David's mother declared that this was not possible. She told Dr. Franklin that David had taken oxycodone briefly after surgery. Dr. Franklin responded that the test suggested more recent ingestion and indicated that today's events had been caused by a drug overdose. The narcotics David had ingested caused severe respiratory depression and a respiratory arrest during sleep when his breathing was most vulnerable.

The fact that this event occurred in the morning hours was no coincidence. The physiologic changes of sleep render narcotics users very vulnerable to the depressant effect on control of breathing in the medulla oblongata. It was likely that David stopped breathing soon before his father found him. After he stopped breathing, his oxygen level dropped, his CO_2 level rose, and within minutes his store of oxygen was depleted, and his heart stopped. Although his heart function had returned to normal following resuscitation, it was evident that David's brain had been deprived of oxygen long enough to cause significant injury,

Would David's brain recover as his heart had? Brain cells are especially vulnerable to a decrease of oxygen. When the brain is without oxygen supply for more than a few minutes, permanent brain injury often occurs. Dr. Franklin discussed the hospital's hypothermia protocol with David's parents. There was compelling evidence that cooling the body for twenty-four hours could improve David's chance of recovery of brain function.

Of course, David's parents had no hesitation. Anything to improve David's chance for a favorable neurological outcome was worth trying. Dr. Franklin expressed some optimism, given David's youth and otherwise healthy body. David's parents never left the bedside. The nurses provided a cot so that his parents could rest. Peter and Rebecca slept off and on through the night. At least one of them always held David's hand and whispered loving thoughts. David's two brothers, from out of town, were on their way. At 6:00 A.M., Dr. Franklin returned to give an update on David's condition.

Peter and Rebecca were praying that their beloved son would open his eyes and smile. Their concern was heightened when Dr. Franklin indicated that he would request consultation by a neurologist. Dr. Colby, the attending neurologist, was a tall, thin, bespectacled physician who sported a bow tie. He was straightforward and not so much the warm and fuzzy type.

Later that evening, Dr. Colby completed his exam. He explained to David's parents that a CT scan of the head performed earlier that day showed evidence of severe anoxic brain injury. In laymen's terms, he explained that David's brain had suffered from a lack of oxygen after he stopped breathing. He did, however, give Peter and Rebecca hope and indicated that it was still too soon to tell if David could recover neurological function. Family members took turns holding David's hand and reading to him as he remained comatose. That night, David was placed on continuous EEG monitoring, looking for seizure activity that might be amenable to medical care and possibly explain why he was not waking up.

As each day passed, the prognosis became grimmer. Continuous EEG monitoring showed lack of brain activity while the heart monitor showed normal, regular electrical functioning. The EEG was flat line. David's parents looked for signs of hope but there were none. David failed to open his eyes when asked. He failed to squeeze a hand when family members pleaded for him to do so. Tears flowed from all family members at the bedside. This beautiful shy boy who had developed into a talented athlete was slipping away.

It was my weekend to cover the intensive care unit. Friday, after 5:00 P.M., my four pulmonary/critical care physician colleagues provided a verbal sign-out of patients for evaluation during the weekend. David was one of them. Dr. Franklin was the last to sign out on Friday evening. He reviewed David's clinical presentation and course and indicated that EEG and physical exam were consistent with brain death.

Although people commonly think of death as an irreversible cessation of cardiac pumping, specific criteria leading to the diagnosis of brain death also signify end of life and allow one to pronounce death with a beating heart. These criteria are necessary in an era of mechanical ventilation, which has allowed us to continue to provide oxygen to a beating heart despite the absence of brain function.

To meet the definition of brain death, David would be evaluated by the attending neurologist and undergo an apnea test. Saturday after rounds, I met with Peter and Rebecca. I needed to be sure they understood the events that had transpired. We discussed how the attending neurologist had examined David twice that day and found no evidence of brain activity. David's brain stem, the core of the brain responsible for breathing, showed no evidence of functioning. The neurologist tested for pupillary response to a flashlight, checked for a gag or cough when passing a catheter into the throat, evaluated for corneal reflexes of the eyes upon stimulation with a wisp of tissue paper, and watched for eye movement when cold water was instilled into the ears.

Any response to these provocative measures would suggest ongoing brain stem function. No responses were evident. David remained comatose with no reaction to painful stimulation. His catastrophic brain injury from lack of oxygen had led to widespread death of vital brain cells. No other medical condition was present to explain his neurological condition. The outcome appeared grimmer by the hour. Peter and Rebecca indicated that David had expressed the wish to donate his organs upon his death.

This terrific athlete who had been bullied in his younger days had remained sensitive and generous. The Gift of Life organization was contacted and two nurses who had dedicated their careers to organ transplantation arrived to meet with the family. As my hand squeezed Peter's, I revealed that I had children and grandchildren and that I could not imagine what he was going through. Tears flowed from the eyes of Peter and Rebecca.

I explained the procedure for an apnea test. I discussed that, although the EEG was flat line and a CT scan showed severe anoxic brain injury, and that multiple neurological exams showed no response, the final test to declare brain death with certainty was an apnea test. David's parents said they understood and proceeded to the intensive care unit waiting room.

I assembled our team of ICU residents, nurses, and respiratory therapists. Prior to beginning, all members of the medical team had the opportunity to express any questions or concerns regarding the test or David's condition. A period of silence followed. I assigned a task to each member of the medical team. We increased David's inspired oxygen and subsequently checked an arterial blood gas. We wanted to make sure David's blood was carrying an extra reserve of oxygen from the ventilator and that his carbon dioxide was normal prior to disconnecting the tube from the ventilator. The breathing tube would remain in David's trachea connected to a source of oxygen but no longer connected to the ventilator that actively pumped in oxygen and removed carbon dioxide.

The resident was instructed to stare at David's chest and abdomen and watch intently for any signs of breathing. We hoped for a signal that somehow David's brain stem was still intact and able to deliver a message to breathe. The intern served as scribe and recorded vital signs every minute. I instructed the respiratory therapist to disconnect the ventilator from the tube and thread an oxygen catheter down the breathing tube. We did not want to deprive David of oxygen during his test.

Indeed, if his oxygen level dropped during the study, that would be an indication to stop the testing. Breath holding in an awake individual leads to a buildup of carbon dioxide in the blood. This causes profound discomfort and serves as a strong stimulus to the brain stem to send electrical impulses to the muscles of breathing.

We hoped that with disconnection of the ventilator, David's rising carbon dioxide levels would lead to respiratory effort. Minutes seemed like hours after David was disconnected from the ventilator. As each minute passed, I also stared at

David's chest, abdomen, and neck, looking and hoping and praying that in this athletic youth there was still a chance that brain activity would respond to a rising level of carbon dioxide. I had given instructions to the team that the test would be stopped immediately, and David would be reconnected to the ventilator if his oxygen level dropped, his heart monitor showed instability, or if he demonstrated any effort to breathe.

At minute five, there was still no evidence of respiratory effort. We obtained another arterial blood gas from the catheter in David's wrist. The results returned quickly and demonstrated an increase in carbon dioxide. This elevation in the volatile acid produced through cellular metabolism reflected absence of breathing on David's part. Ordinarily, in a patient with an intact functioning brain stem, elevation of carbon dioxide is a potent stimulus to breathe. The fact that David showed no respiratory effort at five minutes was very discouraging. At ten minutes, another arterial blood gas was obtained. David still showed no evidence of respiratory effort.

The testing was concluded, and David was reconnected to the ventilator. The arterial blood gas results returned and revealed that his carbon dioxide level had risen by greater than 20-mmHg (millimeters of mercury). This was indeed a positive apnea test. David showed no respiratory effort despite an elevation in carbon dioxide from a normal level to greater than a 20-mmHg increase. This clearly supported what we already strongly suspected. David's brain had ceased to perform its most basic task. The very core of his brain stem that controlled breathing would no longer function to sustain life.

I declared David dead. Although the discomfort of declaring death in the presence of a beating heart may be quite profound, a learned body of physicians, ethicists, and lawmakers has established that declaration of death is appropriate when all criteria of brain death have been unequivocally satisfied.

As I left the intensive care unit, I felt great sadness. This young man's life had been cut short. Peter and Rebecca were deprived of their beautiful son, and his brothers were deprived of their best friend. As I entered the waiting room, my appearance was met with loud cries. No words were necessary on my part. David's family looked at my saddened facial expression and knew their son was gone.

I explained that organ donation, in keeping with David's wishes, would soon proceed but first I would evaluate David's airways with a fiberoptic bronchoscope for any evidence of infection. As a pulmonologist, I had performed this procedure more than a thousand times to diagnose disease and implement treatment. All prior procedures were in living, breathing patients. I had never performed a postmortem bronchoscopy.

As I passed the bronchoscope into David's airway, I glanced at the monitor as he was still connected to the ventilator and his heart was still beating. We wanted to ensure continued delivery of oxygen to all his organs so they would remain viable for their recipients. I wondered who would have the good fortune of receiving these young healthy lungs? Who would receive this beautiful beating heart of a lion? Who would receive the kidneys of this champion? Though David was too young to die, he left a legacy so that others would live on because of his generosity.

After I completed my evaluation of his beautifully preserved airways, he was transported to the operating room, where a team of surgeons and nurses awaited his arrival for the extraction of his organs. As soon as his organs were removed, they were to be flown to multiple individuals awaiting David's most generous, precious gifts.

In 1967, a landmark medical development forever changed the landscape of critical care and death determination. With the first heart transplant, performed by Dr. Christiaan Barnard, came the growing need for vital organs for transplantation. The paradox of procuring functioning organs from dead individuals fueled ethical and religious debates on how to guide the medical community in this process.

The following year, the Harvard Ad Hoc Committee proposed that an individual could be declared dead at the point in time when irreversible cessation of the entire brain was established. This revolutionary concept allowed a diagnosis of death in a patient with a beating heart. This event is only relevant in a patient sustained by mechanical ventilation. In the person breathing spontaneously who develops total absence of

135

brain function, cessation of nerve transmission to the diaphragm quickly follows. This leads to cessation of breathing, loss of circulating oxygen, and cardiac arrest with diagnosis of death by traditional means.

In 1981, the President's Commission for the Study of Ethical Problems in Medicine and Biomedical and Behavioral Research published "Defining Death: Medical, Legal, and Ethical Issues in the Determination of Death." This led to the development of the Uniform Determination of Death Act (UDDA) that states, "An individual who has sustained either 1) irreversible cessation of circulatory and respiratory function, or 2) irreversible cessation of all function of the entire brain, including the brain stem, is dead. A determination of death must be made in accordance with accepted standards."

Since the development of the UDDA, every state in the United States has adopted a version of this approach to death determination. In 2008, the U.S. President's Council on Bioethics reinforced this approach: "This body continues to endorse the concept that total brain failure serves as criterion for declaring death." Some states indicate that a physician may not declare death based upon neurological criteria if such a determination would be inconsistent with the patient's personal religious beliefs. Although these definitions of death, including brain death, assist the medical providers in the process of organ donation, the physician must be aware of the laws of the state within which he or she practices.

It also must be clearly stated that coma from a persistent vegetative state affecting the cerebral cortex and interfering with cognitive functioning is not the same as brain death. The definition of brain death includes cessation of the core brain structure known as the brain stem.

To declare brain death and, therefore, cessation of the functioning brain stem, widely established criteria used to demonstrate with certainty absence of function of this core structure must be met before the physician may declare that end of life has occurred. Once this event is documented by the attending physician, organ procurement may then legally and ethically proceed in an effort to sustain the life of others.

20

7th Inning Stretch

While watching a Phillies game, I began to experience a presleep sensation of body relaxation in my comfortable recliner. I approached that point of ambivalence: whether to turn off the TV and get into bed or push to watch another inning. That internal debate took place on many nights.

I have loved watching and playing sports since early childhood. With two older brothers and a younger sister, sports had become an important part of our lives. As a medical student and then as a physician, playing competitive sports was vital to my work-life balance. Activity in sports such as basketball or tennis always seemed to bring me back to a feeling of tranquility, a sensation that was easily disrupted by the intensity of medical decision making.

Work-life balance and avoidance of burnout were never discussed in my early years of practice. The profession has finally realized that its future survival depends on greater focus on humanity and compassion, not only for our patients but also for ourselves. As doctors in American society, we are afforded great privileges. The cost of these privileges is a higher incidence of depression, burnout, alcoholism, drug dependency, and death by suicide. Seeing our patients endure great suffering and dealing with the uncertainties of clinical medicine are major contributing factors.

It was Friday night. Weekends off are very important for physicians and other healthcare providers. It gives us a chance to recharge our depleted batteries. Recharging and maintaining work-life balance were essential factors in avoiding burnout and compassion fatigue.

By this point in my career, I had been afforded the opportunity to have most weekends off. However, this was my weekend on call to cover for the other physicians in our pulmonary/critical care section. The practice of physician cross coverage is essential so that each of us has time to devote to family, friends, personal growth, and self-care.

My responsibilities for the weekend included caring for hospitalized patients, responding to consults, fielding calls from outpatients, coordinating transfers from outside hospitals, and teaching the interns and residents on rounds.

I had the good fortune of practicing in a teaching hospital staffed twenty-four hours a day, seven days a week by high-quality interns and residents. These young doctors are in the early stages of their medical training. In exchange for the teaching that an attending physician such as myself provides, these young physicians serve as our eyes and ears while we attending physicians evaluate other patients or are at home sleeping or enjoying the company of our loved ones.

I had served as an intern and a resident more than thirty years ago and was quite sympathetic to their stressful lives characterized by long work hours, sleepless nights, and lack of work-life balance. The well-established hierarchy in medical training dictated that patients were treated both day and night by young physicians supervised by older, more experienced ones. The dynamic nature of medical illness requires serial evaluations to address changing conditions. It was this dynamic of medical illness that made working as a pulmonary/critical care physician challenging and stressful, while rewarding and interesting.

When I was on call, most situations could be handled over the telephone through conversations with residents and interns. I always knew that at any minute an emergency could arise, requiring my direct involvement by telephone or my return to the hospital.

At 10:00 P.M., my cell phone rang. I immediately recognized the digital display of the hospital emergency room number, a number I had known for decades, a number that elicited a highly charged emotional response and a surge of catecholamines (stress response). My pre-slumber relaxed state was quickly replaced by a fully conscious hypervigilant one. My fight or flight response, as in all mammals, had developed to prepare for battle.

Watching this baseball game would have to wait. After I got a call that evening, I knew that something significantly more important demanded my attention. I first learned of Donnie that night when I was called by the emergency department physician. His dwindling supply of delicate air sacs had to work harder to compensate. Ongoing inhalation of tobacco chemicals had destroyed his lungs as acid burns away tissue paper. Ultimately, his progressive loss of lung function led to the daily experience of significant shortness of breath.

Donnie had been cautioned on multiple occasions that his smoking would certainly lead to progressive deterioration in his breathing. Despite trying various pharmacologic interventions to assist him with smoking cessation, these measures proved to no avail. Nicotine addiction was too powerful for Donnie to overcome.

Donnie's breathing difficulties initially were mild, but his condition progressed to the point where walking across the room was a major challenge. His pulmonologist, an expert in diseases of the lungs, ordered pulmonary function testing that confirmed that Donnie suffered from severe COPD related to many years of inhaling harmful chemicals packed into cigarettes—perfectly symmetrical cylinders of death.

Inhalers, also known as bronchodilators, led to minimal improvement in his breathing. As Donnie became more vulnerable to life-threatening pneumonia, he was given a pneumonia vaccine and received a yearly flu shot. He worked as a bartender; he loved chatting and was an excellent listener. He enjoyed providing advice to guests as they smoked and drank. The late-night hours suited him well and were in sync with his sleep-wake circadian rhythm. He enjoyed a 4:00 A.M. bedtime and usually slept until noon.

Bartending exposed Donnie to an occupational hazard. In addition to his two-pack-a-day habit, daily eight-hour shifts with secondhand smoke exposure combined to progressively destroy his delicate lungs and contribute to what has become one of the major causes of death worldwide: chronic obstructive pulmonary disease, more commonly known as COPD. Most of Donnie's tiny air sacs, known as alveoli, had been destroyed over the decades. His lungs could no longer function to deliver oxygen and excrete carbon dioxide as efficiently as they had in his younger days.

Nancy was the emergency room attending physician on the evening I received the call. I had worked with her for many years, and in fact, we had served as interns together. Our conversations started with questions about our children and our spouses. After a moment of greetings, Nancy summarized Donnie's presentation. Communication through doctor-to-doctor telephone conversation plays a crucial role in the practice of medicine. Important decisions are made based on brief discussions. The course of these discussions typically follows a format learned in medical school and refined with practice and experience.

Nancy communicated that Donnie was a patient followed by one of my colleagues for whom I was covering. He was described as a sixty-eight-year-old male with a history of chronic obstructive pulmonary disease and congestive heart failure presenting to the emergency room with increasing shortness of breath with activity. His shortness of breath progressed to the point where he was having difficulty breathing at rest. He denied chest pain, cough, sputum production, or fevers.

On exam, Donnie was breathing more rapidly than normal with a respiratory rate of twenty-six breaths per minute. He was using accessory neck muscles to supplement the ineffective functioning of his diaphragm. His chest exam revealed bilateral wheezes. His heart exam demonstrated a regular rhythm but was beating rapidly at 120 beats per minute. His legs showed swelling in both ankles, a reflection of backflow of fluid from the heart.

Nancy noted that his chest X-ray displayed fluid in the lungs. The EKG showed no signs of a heart attack. Arterial blood gas demonstrated a decrease in blood pH, an increase in carbon dioxide, and a reduced oxygen level.

Nancy's review of Donnie's presentation was very succinct and gave a clear picture of his respiratory issues and severity of disease. Although not at his bedside evaluating him in person, I felt comfortable with Nancy's assessment. After our discussion, we decided to provide nebulizer treatments with bronchodilators and systemic steroids to diminish the inflammation of his disease-narrowed bronchial tubes.

We also discussed placing Donnie on a noninvasive ventilator. This miraculous device allows for delivery of oxygen and excretion of carbon dioxide without placing a breathing tube in the patient's throat. In patients with a COPD exacerbation, intervention with this device has proved lifesaving for many.

We discussed that if Donnie deteriorated despite these interventions, a breathing tube would be placed for attachment to a ventilator. Although typically, and in keeping with Occam's Razor (that the simplest explanation is the most likely), one disease process is responsible for a patient's specific clinical presentation, sometimes two or more disease processes were simultaneously involved. The challenge was to determine the relative contribution of each and then to initiate the most effective and least harmful therapy.

In Donnie's case, he had both COPD and congestive heart failure. These conditions may act synergistically as they lead to progressive respiratory failure and possibly death without appropriate intervention. Donnie's COPD was caused by many years of smoking cigarettes and exposure to secondhand smoke. Cigarette smoke, when inhaled, causes white blood cells in the lungs to release a protein known as elastase. This protein punches holes in tiny delicate air sacs over a period of many years. The cumulative effect is permanent destruction of enough air sacs to make breathing a great challenge.

Most of the time, we take for granted the vital functioning of our breathing and the great gift that it is. If lungs become significantly impaired because of progressive disease, the breathing rate often increases to compensate and maintain delivery of oxygen and adequate excretion of carbon dioxide. Patients with COPD frequently experience a transient deterioration known as an exacerbation due to a respiratory tract infection. The inflammation of the airways caused by infection leads to a temporary worsening of the narrowed airways. It was as if Donnie were breathing through a straw.

Donnie's situation also was more complicated because of his coexistent congestive heart failure. His heart was unable to pump blood efficiently to his vital organs. This deterioration in heart function led to a backup of fluid in his lungs. With Donnie's COPD exacerbation causing a low oxygen level, this may have triggered a deterioration of his heart function by depriving the cells of the heart the valuable oxygen needed to contract.

We decided to treat Donnie for both an exacerbation of COPD and for deterioration in his congestive heart failure. While waiting for nebulizer treatments, steroids, and the noninvasive ventilator to improve his COPD exacerbation, we gave intravenous Lasix, a potent diuretic. This medicine increases urine output by turning on the spigot in the kidneys, leading to total decrease in body fluid and drying out of the lungs. We hoped that as his COPD was treated and fluid left his lungs, Donnie's breathing would return to baseline so he could survive this crisis.

Nancy and I both agreed that Donnie was not sick enough to require admission to the intensive care unit but was too sick to go to a regular hospital floor. We admitted him to an intermediate critical care unit where nurses could monitor his progress closely and notify an intern if any deterioration necessitating transfer to the intensive care unit developed. We understood that this was a dynamic situation and that changes may occur, requiring reevaluation and an adjustment in decision making.

After finishing my discussion with Nancy, I kissed my wife goodnight, rested my head on a comfortable pillow, and hoped for quick entry into dreamland. That feeling of sleepiness I had experienced while watching the Phillies game had been replaced by intense focus brought on by a catecholamine surge. Discussing patients with critical illness consistently led to a state of extreme alertness at any time, day or night. The stakes were too high to pursue clinical decision making in any other mental state.

The challenge tonight was to change gears quickly after the discussion and turn off the switch so sleep onset was not delayed. As I aged and felt increasingly more comfortable with decision making, turning off the switch came more easily.

At 3:00 A.M., my cell phone awakened me. I immediately wondered whether Donnie had deteriorated. Had I relied too much on the evaluation of other physicians? Had I overlooked other potential contributing factors such as blood clots? Should I have gone into the hospital to evaluate him personally? Would I be informed that Donnie died? These are the questions concerned and conscientious healthcare providers ask themselves in the middle of the night. These are the uncertainties all healthcare providers, whether as novice or mature practitioner, face while caring for critically ill patients.

Although it is reasonable and appropriate to reexamine and reflect on clinical decisions, it is counterproductive to assume the worst. Assuming that Donnie had deteriorated due to an error in my judgment that would culminate in disapproval and shaming from colleagues is a dangerous, dysfunctional cognitive distortion. So many physicians suffer in silence from overwhelming feelings of guilt, fear, and self-doubt, magnified by distorted thinking contributing to melancholy, clinical depression, and suicide.

Dr. Aaron Beck, regarded as the pioneer of cognitive behavioral therapy, teaches that distorted reasoning such as jumping to negative conclusions without evidence to support such assumptions contributes to feelings of sadness and depression. It is often a distorted interpretation of an event rather than the event itself that leads to negative thoughts and feelings.

Even if Donnie had deteriorated, it did not necessarily mean that my judgment was faulty. But what if Donnie's clinical condition worsened due to an error in my decision making? What if he died because we had not made the correct diagnosis? After all, we clinicians are human, and humans make mistakes. Would I endure unbearable emotional pain from contributing to the loss of a human life precipitated by a bad medical decision—an unfortunate medical error depriving a family of their loved one? Would my colleagues think less of me and avoid my opinions in consultation in the future?

Although we must never be complacent, to maintain a healthy emotional state it is essential for all healthcare providers to anticipate and accept the greatly feared possibility of human error causing or contributing to a patient's demise. Rather than jumping to unhealthy distorted conclusions in response, it is essential to learn and evolve to prevent future errors when similar situations arise. No clinician can know everything. Perfection is beyond reach for us mere mortals.

Rather than pursuing the downward spiral characterized by feelings of extreme guilt related to an actual or perceived error, the healthier approach involves self-compassion while engaging in lifelong learning, consultation with colleagues, and serial reevaluations of a patient's clinical status. The insightful clinician practices with flexibility and integrates new information followed by adjustments in diagnosis and treatment accordingly.

A medical error resulting in death is a devastating experience for the patient's loved ones. Many questions inevitably surface. The family of the decedent must be approached with compassion and transparency. After an honest explanation of the events that transpired, an apology is in order. Furthermore, a detailed discussion of specific plans to prevent such an event in the future should follow. This process, with humility and honesty, will help facilitate the healing process for both family and provider. For the clinician who caused or contributed to a fatal medical error, the emotional impact will be quite significant and undoubtedly have a lasting effect.

To support healthcare providers with learning and growth from unfortunate patient outcomes, Morbidity and Mortality conferences are convened on a regular basis in our institution. These peer-protected sessions allow physicians to discuss adverse events, including death. Open discussions, without fear of retribution, serve as an opportunity to develop as clinicians and improve the decision-making process. As positive outcomes are never a certainty in medicine, errors may be identified to enhance the likelihood of survival of future patients who encounter similar situations.

As it turned out, the call was unrelated to Donnie. Our Health System Transfer Center was on the line. Bill, the nurse at the Transfer Center, informed me of a request from an outside hospital to transfer a patient from their intensive care unit to ours. Our hospital, as part of the University of Pennsylvania Health System, reviews requests for transfers at any hour.

The nurse connected me with Dr. Eldridge, a physician from a small hospital intensive care unit approximately 100 miles away. He asked if we could accept a patient whose kidneys were failing and in need of dialysis. They did not have a nephrologist in their institution to provide this lifesaving service. After determining that the patient was reasonably stable based upon vital signs and electrolytes, I accepted the patient in transfer. Dr. Eldridge expressed his gratitude as he and I certainly were aligned in our interests for the well-being of this patient.

As Dr. Eldridge arranged for transport by ambulance, I notified our intensive care unit resident on call to expect the patient's arrival within several hours. I then went back to sleep. As an attending at a teaching hospital, my sleep was disrupted far less frequently than physicians practicing in community hospitals without interns and residents.

My alarm clock sounded at 7:30 A.M. I showered, ate breakfast, and walked down the street to the hospital to begin rounds. Two years earlier, my wife and I had left the suburbs for city life. Our children had their own children and the time had come for us to downsize. The days of long commuting were over. I could walk to the hospital and arrive within ten minutes. ICU rounds started at 8:30 A.M. and were completed three hours later.

After a quick lunch, I went to evaluate Donnie in his hospital room. He appeared well and said he felt great. His shortness of breath had resolved and I developed a feeling of great joy for him. Although I needed to guard against the emotional roller coaster that was too closely tied to patient outcome, I felt great happiness from a positive clinical response.

My rounding that Saturday ended at 6:00 P.M. I met my wife for dinner at a local restaurant and spent a quiet evening at home watching one of our Netflix favorites. That night was a peaceful one without sleep disruption. ICU rounds on Sunday started again at 8:30 A.M. Rounds were often interrupted by phone calls from outpatients at home, interns requesting consults, nurses with management questions, or intensive care unit admissions.

While we were reviewing the course of a patient on a ventilator in the ICU, Dr. Edwards, a cardiologist, walked toward us. With her typical mellow demeanor, she told me Donnie was now having trouble breathing and should be transferred to the intensive care unit. This surprised me greatly as Donnie had been improving so nicely when I evaluated him less than twenty-four hours earlier. This was the dynamic nature of critical illness.

Without hesitation, we headed to the intermediate critical care unit to evaluate Donnie. The journey took only several minutes as we climbed the steps to the fourth floor. With each step, I pondered why Donnie had improved and then worsened. Would we be able to determine quickly which intervention should be instituted to prevent further decline and possibly death?

Immediately upon arrival, it was clear that Donnie was having considerable trouble breathing. I asked one of the residents to count Donnie's respiratory rate. While I bent over to listen to Donnie's heart and lungs with my stethoscope, I instructed the nurse to obtain a STAT chest X-ray, electrocardiogram, and arterial blood gas. This triad of testing is routine for any patient in respiratory distress. The information from these tests routinely proves to be invaluable in decision making.

The exam revealed that Donnie had good breath sounds bilaterally and was not wheezing. His heart sounds were regular and fast. Donnie was sucking in air and unable to complete full sentences without gasping. He told me that he had been feeling well until he was awakened from sleep with shortness of breath. A nebulizer treatment with albuterol, a bronchodilator, did not help.

I knew we had to act quickly. The resident called out the number thirty-five; Donnie's breath rate was twice normal. By now, Ms. Hargrove, the respiratory therapist, was by my side. I asked her to place Donnie on his noninvasive ventilator. I turned to the nurse and instructed her to call anesthesia in anticipation of the likely need for placement of a breathing tube in his windpipe. The resident who had called out the number thirty-five was puzzled, as if he wanted to ask, why anesthesia?

I turned to Donnie and his two daughters standing by his side. I held Donnie's hand and explained that if his breathing did not improve quickly on the noninvasive ventilator device, we would request that anesthesia place a breathing tube through his mouth into his windpipe to provide full ventilatory support. Donnie nodded in full understanding and his daughters agreed.

I believed there was a good chance that the use of a noninvasive ventilator could help us avoid intubation with an endotracheal tube, but I did not want to take any chance that Donnie would deteriorate further with a delay in calling anesthesia, possibly leading to a worse outcome. It was clear that things could worsen quickly and without much notice. Donnie could decline and develop full cardiopulmonary arrest. I then stepped back and asked myself: why was this happening? Why did Donnie improve significantly and then subsequently get worse? My clinical suspicion was that Donnie's congestive heart failure had worsened during the early morning hours of sleep.

Although, as a relatively thin man with a normal-sized neck circumference, Donnie did not have the typical body habitus of obstructive sleep apnea, this was a consideration. Patients with obstructive sleep apnea stop breathing repeatedly during sleep. It was possible that Donnie had undiagnosed obstructive sleep apnea that triggered a recurrence of his congestive heart failure as his airway closed repeatedly while sleeping, causing a drop in his oxygen level.

I asked the nurse to give Donnie 40 mg of IV Lasix. This potent diuretic could improve breathing very quickly if congestive heart failure was the cause of his deterioration. Soon after Lasix was infused, Donnie's bedside urinal began to fill, and his clinical condition started to improve. His respiratory rate normalized, and he no longer appeared to be gasping for air.

It was quickly apparent that Donnie did not require intubation. The anesthesia team arrived and were awaiting our instructions. As I glanced at the resident who had seemed to question why I summoned the team, I turned my attention to the anesthesiologist and thanked her for responding quickly, apologized for any inconvenience, and indicated that the patient was improving, and therefore would not require intubation at this time. The anesthesiologist smiled and said no problem. She told us to call if they were needed.

The anesthesia team returned to their on-call quarters, and we wheeled Donnie into the intensive care unit. Although he was improving greatly, we wanted to monitor him more closely and resume ICU rounds. There were several other patients we needed to evaluate.

Rounds that day finished by 5:00 P.M. My last patient of the day in a regular floor bed, suspected of having tuberculosis. I donned an N95 mask as the patient was in respiratory isolation. He was improving on treatment. After authoring my last note in the electronic medical records, I joined my wife at home for dinner. After dinner, I contacted my physician colleagues for whom I had covered to review events of the weekend. They would each return Monday morning, fully charged, rested, and ready to resume care of their patients.

I slept well that night. Monday morning, I returned to work with a sense of great satisfaction. Although I had seen many patients over that weekend, none were as memorable as Donnie. I never saw Donnie again but heard that he was discharged from the hospital three days later. From time to time, I remember Donnie. And I recall the medical team of doctors including interns and residents, nurses, and respiratory therapists who were at his bedside that Sunday morning working together for one sole purpose, that of helping another human being breathe more easily.

21

Obstructive Sleep Apnea

In 2020, a year nobody will ever forget, while awaiting notification of a possible redeployment to the ICU to care for patients critically ill with COVID-19 infection, I performed the important task of telemedicine. This modern technological advance allows physicians to connect with outpatients without risk of direct contact. Social distancing became the norm to decrease the spread of the deadly virus.

My goal was to keep my patients healthy at home. As I walked down the street to my Center City office, I noticed an occasional pedestrian, masked and gloved. Upon entering my office building where I practice, I was greeted by a nurse who placed a sticker on my ID card and checked my temperature with a thermal sensor placed several inches from my forehead. If a fever were detected, I would be sent home.

Within seconds, I was given the okay to proceed to my ninth-floor office. The three elevators, which were normally filled, were empty and punctual. I arrived in my office after greeting Jennifer, our practice nurse. She and I were both wearing masks and kept the obligatory six feet from each other.

After logging onto my computer, I checked for urgent e-mails and hospital updates. My courageous younger pulmonary colleagues were caring for ten patients on ventilators afflicted with COVID-19. Many of these patients were likely to die. Colleagues caring for these patients could potentially be exposed to high viral loads generated from aerosolized particles as the ventilators dispersed virus-laden exhaled air into the room's atmosphere. Hopefully, the personal protective equipment, including masks, gloves, gowns, and goggles, in conjunction with filters on the ventilator exhalation tubes, would protect them from this deadly pathogen.

Our hospital's redeployment protocol was structured to protect older physicians like me, who were at greater risk, while drawing on our years of experience through telemedicine. At the same time, I had made it clear to my younger colleagues that I was available if they became ill or needed backup. I had cared for many patients as a younger pulmonologist during the AIDS epidemic and was ready to provide my services to those with COVID-19 should the need arise.

I surveyed my outpatient schedule of new patient visits. One of the names looked quite familiar. It was not uncommon for a patient to resurface many years after prior care. Over more than thirty years of clinical practice, I have developed a following of patients suffering from various respiratory conditions. Some saw me regularly without missing an appointment. Others resurfaced after a brief or long hiatus.

———

I had first met Melanie ten years earlier when she weighed over 400 pounds. Obesity has become an epidemic in our nation. This deadly medical condition has especially plagued the urban poor community where fast-food restaurants can be seen on almost every corner.

As Melanie's weight increased, the soft tissues in her throat enlarged and compromised her upper airway. With skeletal muscle relaxation during sleep, her airway was repeatedly obstructed for thirty to sixty seconds. This is known as obstructive sleep apnea. In an extremely adaptive response, evolution has equipped all of us with a brain stem that is highly responsive to a drop in oxygen and an increase in carbon dioxide following repeated airway closure due to obstructive sleep apnea.

The medulla oblongata at the core of the brain stem contains a cluster of cells known as the Pre-Bötzinger Complex. These and other cells, in response to elevation in carbon dioxide and drops in oxygen, send patterned signals down the neural pathways to the muscles of breathing. Progressively powerful signals ultimately lead to reopening of the obstructed airway.

This highly regulated neural response kept Melanie from dying of suffocation. As Melanie stopped breathing more than 100 times per hour during sleep, each apneic event was followed by a brief reopening of the airway, just long enough for her to suck in oxygen and expel carbon dioxide. The cumulative effect of repeated drops in oxygen over many years had taken its toll. When I first met Melanie, she was critically ill in the intensive care unit as she had developed a failing heart with a backup of fluid in her lungs and legs. She was in congestive heart failure. Her cognitive functioning had declined due to repeated bouts of oxygen depletion and sleep deprivation.

A pressurized device known as nasal CPAP, used to keep the airway open during sleep, is highly effective for most people with obstructive sleep apnea, but Melanie had not tolerated this approach. After a discussion with Melanie and her family, we agreed to proceed with tracheostomy. Her surgeon placed a two-inch incision in her neck so that a curved six-inch tube could be placed into her windpipe. This device was placed below her vocal cords to preserve her speech. As the recurrent nocturnal airway obstruction Melanie had been experiencing was in the back of her throat, the trach tube opening lower in her windpipe would serve as a bypass to allow oxygen to enter her lungs and carbon dioxide to leave with each inhalation and exhalation during sleep. She would be able to talk without difficulty by placing a cap on the trach opening during the day and would simply uncap the trach at night to prevent airway obstruction while she slept.

After the tracheostomy had been completed, I evaluated Melanie in the intensive care unit where she was recovering. As I opened the curtain that surrounded her hospital bed, I assumed a routine post-op check would follow. I had no idea that a brief powerful human connection would occur. With the head of Melanie's bed comfortably elevated at approximately 45 degrees, I could see tears streaming from her eyes and an ear-to-ear smile. Tears in the ICU generally meant great sadness from news such as impending death. These were undoubtedly joyous tears.

Although the trach incision had brought mild local discomfort, the relief of airway obstruction had liberated Melanie from the traumatic recurrent experience of airway suffocation during sleep. As I extended my hand, Melanie grasped it with great fervor as she spoke the words every physician craves: "Thank you, doctor."

That special moment with Melanie reminded me of the extreme privilege afforded to me as a healthcare provider caring for others and the great meaning and purpose of a life as a physician—the great honor of joining a profession like no other. Although many years of sacrifice had culminated in this magical spiritual moment, I knew that the path had been well worth it. I savored this moment, then and again as the memory resurfaced from time to time.

Years later, when Melanie appeared on my computer screen during a telehealth visit, I knew she looked familiar. During our conversation, Melanie informed me that she had undergone weight loss surgery and had lost more than 100 pounds. Although her obstructive sleep apnea persisted, it had improved sufficiently to allow removal of her tracheostomy tube. She was now able to tolerate a CPAP device to treat her less life-threatening sleep-related apneic events.

———

It is estimated that 25 million adults in the United States suffer from obstructive sleep apnea, arguably the most common breathing disorder. This is well over 10 percent of all adults in the country. The rising number of patients afflicted with this condition is, in part, attributed to the obesity epidemic.

While awake, as we generate negative intrathoracic pressure to suck in air, the tendency for the upper airway to collapse is opposed by muscles that keep the airway open.

During sleep, however, with skeletal muscle relaxation, this opposing force to maintain upper airway patency is diminished in everyone.

A non-obese patient may develop obstructive sleep apnea through excessive upper airway relaxation in combination with airway abnormalities such as enlarged tonsils, nasal obstruction, micrognathia (a small lower jaw), or retrognathia (a set-back lower jaw, as with an overbite). Deposition of excessive fat in the upper airways of the obese patient further predisposes the patient to repetitive partial or complete upper airway collapse during sleep.

Collapse of the airway during sleep may last ten seconds or significantly longer. In association with these episodes of airway collapse, oxygen levels may drop quite significantly. In the patient with an intact brain stem, not impaired by the presence of narcotics or benzodiazepines, the brain stem will typically respond to the associated drop in oxygen level and collapsed airway. The brain stem sends a very strong signal to the airway muscles with resultant opening of the airway and resumption of airflow and, therefore, oxygen delivery.

This cyclical process may result in hundreds of apneas per night and may go undetected for many years. Without treatment, patients are at increased risk for stroke, congestive heart failure, heart attack, atrial fibrillation, premature death, as well as traffic accidents caused by falling asleep. There is some evidence that of the three phenotypes of obstructive sleep apnea—the excessively sleepy patient, the patient with difficulty maintaining sleep, and the asymptomatic patient—cardiovascular risk is primarily associated with the subset of patients with excessive daytime sleepiness.

Imaging of the brain in patients with severe untreated obstructive sleep apnea has demonstrated a decline in white matter fibers. This correlates with a drop in cognitive functioning. These anatomic abnormalities may be reversible with treatment of the obstructive sleep apnea. Untreated obstructive sleep apnea is also associated with Alzheimer's disease.

The advent of CPAP in 1981 by Colin Sullivan revolutionized treatment and provides a nonsurgical approach for most patients. This device gently blows air through the nasal passage and splints the airway open so that it does not collapse during sleep. It is highly effective and can greatly improve the quality of life of a patient suffering from untreated obstructive sleep apnea. A reduction in excessive daytime sleepiness often quickly follows initiation of CPAP treatment. In addition to enhanced quality of life, there is evidence of decreased cardiovascular risk, decreased risk of car crashes, and decreased risk of diabetes mellitus.

For patients who are overweight, weight loss, either through diet or bariatric surgery, may lead to considerable clinical improvement and often resolution of obstructive sleep apnea. Patients who do not tolerate CPAP or wish for an alternative may benefit from an oral appliance that leads to protrusion of the mandible to maintain airway patency. Surgical interventions, including tonsillectomy, repair of a deviated septum, nasal turbinectomy, mandibular advancement, and maxillary-mandibular osteotomy may be performed. Rarely, in severe life-threatening situations, tracheostomy may be contemplated.

In the morbidly obese hypercapnic patient (too much carbon dioxide in the blood) with severe obstructive sleep apnea/obesity hypoventilation syndrome (low oxygen and high carbon dioxide levels) who is unable to tolerate positive airway pressure therapy, a temporary tracheostomy followed by bariatric (weight loss) surgery may be lifesaving. By surgically removing a significant part of the stomach and leaving a small pouch, the patient suffering from obesity will develop early satiety (feeling full with less food) and may lose one-third of their body weight within a year. This often leads to resolution or at least significant improvement in the life-threatening obstructive sleep apnea. The temporary tracheostomy is often then removed and CPAP is usually better tolerated if it is still deemed to be necessary.

Avoidance of excessive sedation with narcotics and benzodiazepines in the postoperative patient with obstructive sleep apnea is essential. The administration of postoperative narcotics in an undiagnosed obstructive sleep apnea patient may in some cases prove fatal.

In recent years, there has been great enthusiasm for the treatment of a subset of patients by implanting a hypoglossal nerve stimulator. In appropriately selected patients, implantation of this stimulator in the neck can be successfully utilized to treat obstructive sleep apnea.

Our future challenge is to train healthcare providers and the public to recognize the signs and symptoms of obstructive sleep apnea earlier so that treatment may be initiated prior to the development of harmful sequelae such as cardiovascular disease, diabetes, and motor vehicle accidents.

Additionally, earlier treatment may greatly improve the quality of life of those who suffer from excessive daytime sleepiness. Clues that should alert the clinician and the public to the possibility of obstructive sleep apnea include a history of loud disruptive snoring (reported by a bed partner and sometimes denied by the patient), nocturnal gasping, witnessed apneas (such as a spouse seeing another spouse stop breathing momentarily), morning headache, daytime sleepiness, falling asleep while driving, difficult-to-control hypertension, history of atrial fibrillation, stroke, or heart attack. The suspicion is heightened in the overweight individual. However, one should not overlook the possibility of obstructive sleep apnea in the patient of normal body weight.

The purpose of Melanie's appointment was ostensibly to obtain new supplies for her device, but more importantly, allowed us to reunite and reminisce about our highly spiritual moment during her critical illness. At the end of Melanie's visit, we thanked each other. She expressed gratitude that I had helped her through a medical crisis ten years ago. I expressed gratitude for having had that opportunity and for reconnecting with her to relive that special moment.

22

Shared Home, Shared Breaths

After Connie and Jessica were married in Vermont, they spent their honeymoon in Europe. Although each was of modest means, they saved up for the vacation of a lifetime, and did their best not to think about all the work needed on their newly purchased home, built in the 1800s, on a quaint street in Center City, Philadelphia.

Toward the end of the trip, their attention turned to decorating. When they returned home after Labor Day, they realized that they had chosen the perfect time of year to start renovations. The cool fall days allowed them to keep windows open as dust was aerosolized and walls were painted. By wintertime, most of the work had been completed. All that remained was to enjoy their new home and stick to a budget to pay the bills. Connie was a hairdresser and Jessica was an information technology specialist at a nearby hospital. They had met through a mutual friend and it was love at first sight.

Heating this large old house was a costly venture. As winter progressed, they agreed to keep the temperature at a comfortable 68 degrees.

By February, Connie and Jessica both started to experience headaches. Within one week, both noted nausea. Their symptoms were rather mild, and neither was particularly alarmed. Perhaps it was something they ate. Connie spent President's Day weekend with her brother and nieces. She had offered to help babysit. FaceTime kept the newlyweds in close contact over the weekend.

Shared Home, Shared Breaths

When Connie returned to Philadelphia on Tuesday morning, she was concerned that Jessica was not answering her cell phone. This was distinctly unusual. As Connie unlocked the door to her home, she yelled, "hello," knowing that this large old home had 18-inch walls. She shrieked when she found Jessica unresponsive in bed. EMS arrived within minutes and, using a small handheld detector, quickly diagnosed carbon monoxide poisoning.

Connie sat in the ambulance as the paramedic placed an intravenous catheter for fluids and 100 percent oxygen therapy by mask. Although her vital signs were stable, Jessica remained comatose. The ambulance sped off to a large Center City medical center where she would soon be placed in a hyperbaric oxygen chamber to treat her carbon monoxide poisoning.

Connie cried, knowing that her life partner might not survive or ever return to normal cognitive functioning. It quickly became clear that both had been suffering from low levels of carbon monoxide poisoning due to a faulty heater. Further decline in the heater's functioning while Connie was away for the weekend led to Jessica's severe poisoning. Connie had feelings of guilt. Had she not been away, perhaps she could have intervened before Jessica progressed to a comatose state.

Carbon monoxide is a deadly gas by-product of fuel combustion. Without proper venting of heating systems, this insidious odorless gas seeps into the air. Oxygen and carbon monoxide molecules compete for seats on the hemoglobin molecules contained in red blood cells. Carbon monoxide is the big bully that shoves oxygen molecules out of the way and thereby prevents oxygen delivery to cells for energy production. Vitas Gerulaitis, a tennis superstar, died in his sleep at age forty in 1994 while visiting a friend because a faulty pool heater leaked carbon monoxide into the guesthouse. He was breathing contaminated air.

Had Connie returned home an hour later, Jessica likely would have been found dead. Timely intervention with hyperbaric oxygen allowed quick displacement of carbon monoxide from her hemoglobin molecules. Within days, she returned to her normal cognitive and physical functioning.

Jessica and Connie pledged to each other to seek regular professional maintenance for their heating system and to install carbon monoxide detectors.

23

Pulmonary Edema

Frank loved to play blackjack at the Atlantic City casinos. He admits that his losses exceeded total winnings through the years, but the fun and challenge made it worthwhile. His congestive heart failure was generally well controlled with medications if he complied. His daily water pill, known as a diuretic, helped keep fluids out of his legs and, more importantly, out of his lungs. His heart function was impaired but if he adhered to medical recommendations, his quality of life was pretty good.

In addition to his multiple medications, Frank was to weigh himself daily, and contact his cardiologist if he gained more than two pounds in any twenty-four-hour period. Such a weight gain would likely signify fluid retention and a need to increase his water pill. Frank also knew the importance of diet. Excessive sodium from fast food was to be avoided.

As a frequent visitor to the Atlantic City casinos, Frank often received complimentary overnight stays in luxury hotels. It was Labor Day weekend and Frank was on a roll. As his winnings accumulated at the blackjack table, he neglected to take his water pill. Food and drinks were delivered to him free of charge. That night, Frank had trouble staying asleep. He woke up on three occasions acutely short of breath and had to sleep on four pillows to keep his head elevated. It was clear that he was retaining fluid and it was getting redistributed into his lungs while in bed.

In the morning, Frank returned to the blackjack table with his winnings from the night before. After an hour of pushing his luck, he started to develop labored breathing. 911 was called and EMS transported Frank to the local hospital. Upon arrival, Frank appeared ashen, diaphoretic (sweating excessively), tachypneic (breathing rapidly), and at death's door.

The emergency department physician diagnosed pulmonary edema, an accumulation of fluid within the lungs. After initiation of noninvasive ventilation through a mask and administration of IV Lasix, Frank urinated 1,500 cc. This led to some improvement in his breathing. Frank insisted on being transferred to Pennsylvania Hospital where all his physicians knew him well.

It was 2:00 A.M., my cell phone rang and aroused me from a deep sleep. The call was from our Health System Transfer Center which was available twenty-four hours a day seven days a week to accept transfers from smaller hospitals because of special services available in our health system or preexisting relationships between patients and doctors in our institution.

Multiple considerations influenced the decision-making process of whether to accept a patient in transfer emergently. Did we have a service to offer that was not available at the originating hospital? Certainly, if they lacked an intensive care unit bed and we had one, we would accept their patient. Did the patient require a procedure such as emergent dialysis that we could perform but they could not? Did the patient need to be stabilized first to tolerate transfer and not die enroute? Should they transfer the patient at 2:00 A.M. when few providers were in the hospital or would it be best for the patient to wait until after 8:00 A.M.?

These were some issues to consider while speaking to outside physicians requesting assistance with the management of their patients. Moreover, a stable patient who was deemed okay for transfer could destabilize in the hours that followed prior to the actual transfer. I relied on the referring physician for an accurate assessment of the patient's medical condition as well as updates up until the time of transfer.

I raised a concern to the referring physician that Frank could deteriorate in transit and have a cardiopulmonary arrest. I was told by the referring physician that Frank was getting agitated and very adamant about immediate transfer. After careful consideration, being aware that Frank's respiratory status remained tenuous, we decided it would be best for Frank to be transferred but not until an endotracheal tube was placed in his airway for placement on a mechanical ventilator so that he could be stabilized for his journey to our hospital.

Additionally, I requested the referring physician to obtain a chest X-ray and arterial blood gas following placement on the ventilator but before transfer. I wanted added certainty that the patient was adequately stabilized and unlikely to have an adverse event in the ambulance.

Frank arrived at our hospital ICU by 6:00 A.M. By then, he had urinated three liters of fluid and was doing quite well. Soon after his arrival, he was easily liberated from mechanical ventilation. After a twenty-four-hour stay in our ICU, Frank was transferred to a hospital floor.

I met with Frank and we discussed his near-death experience. I reviewed my concerns about his dietary indiscretions and medical noncompliance. Frank did not seem too concerned. We arranged for a consult with a dietitian to review what Frank already knew. We reviewed the importance of adhering to a strict medical regimen and monitoring his daily weight as well as follow-up with his cardiologist. At the end of our discussion, I had a distinct feeling that we would be seeing Frank back in our ICU soon.

24

Blue Patient, Brown Blood

Jonathan was a talented musician. By the age of twelve, he was an accomplished pianist. By age fifteen, he had composed several works that left his music teachers in awe. The decision to attend a renowned school of music after high school graduation was an easy one. Even though he loved playing multiple instruments, conducting became his passion.

Midway through his second year at a prominent school of music, at age twenty, Jonathan started to notice gradually progressive shortness of breath. Initially, he attributed this to deconditioning and lack of exercise. Many of his classmates noticed his panting and wheezing, which became evident after walking a few steps. Jonathan decided to see a physician. It was the first time in many years he needed any medical attention. Fortunately, Student Health was just a few blocks away from his apartment.

It was a Friday afternoon when Jonathan entered the waiting room. As he looked around, he saw several healthy-appearing college-age kids, mostly with sniffles and coughs. He passed the time by working on a musical composition. After a two-hour wait, his turn had come.

A nurse asked Jonathan to follow him back to a typical emergency room–type cubicle. With the curtain drawn, he put on a ragged hospital gown that was clean but ready for replacement. Soon thereafter, a woman in scrubs entered and introduced herself. She was a nurse practitioner who had recently completed her training. To Jonathan, she looked quite young, but her warm smile was reassuring. As Jonathan revealed his history of progressive shortness of breath and decreased ability to climb steps, Ms. Gilliard, the nurse practitioner, ordered a chest X-ray and placed a monitor on his finger. When the monitor revealed that Jonathan's oxygen level was low, she placed him on supplemental oxygen by nasal cannula.

Jonathan could quickly feel the gentle stream of oxygen passing through his nasal passages. He had seen this device many times on television medical shows. His fear began to heighten. What could be causing his depletion of oxygen and his shortness of breath? Was it serious? Was it life-threatening? Ms. Gilliard returned to Jonathan's room to show him his chest X-ray. Despite great advances in technology, this simple, inexpensive film of the chest provided valuable insight into Jonathan's respiratory difficulties. She reviewed with him the finding of pneumonia throughout both lungs and that he would require admission to the hospital. It was safest to transport him by ambulance. Arrangements were made for a direct admission to a regular hospital floor.

Soon after arrival, Jonathan was greeted by Stephanie, a super-friendly medical intern. She had a great gift for communication and putting patients at ease. Stephanie explained to Jonathan that his X-ray was concerning but that his condition was likely treatable and reversible. She did not share her suspicion with Jonathan that he suffered from an infection known as pneumocystis carinii pneumonia. It was in the late 1980s and the AIDS epidemic in Philadelphia was in full swing. She explained that antibiotic therapy would be initiated, and that a lung specialist would drop by later in the day.

When I arrived at Jonathan's bedside, it was evident that his respiratory rate was increased at twenty-four times per minute. He did not appear in acute distress, but his mildly increased work of breathing was readily apparent. I explained to Jonathan that we should perform a procedure known as fiberoptic bronchoscopy to collect samples of fluid from his lungs. Following empiric antibiotics which had been initiated, a confirmation of our suspicion for pneumocystis carinii pneumonia was warranted. If indeed pneumocystis were confirmed, this would be considered an AIDS-defining illness.

The thought of AIDS had crossed Jonathan's mind. Two of his close friends had been diagnosed in the past year. Jonathan was advised to eat nothing after midnight in anticipation of sedation required for his bronchoscopy. The next morning, he was wheeled into the bronchoscopy suite. The anesthesiologist placed an intravenous line in his right hand. After three sequential 1 mg injections of the sedative Versed, Jonathan felt a great sense of calmness. He began to talk about his love for Mozart's great works.

As Jonathan drifted into a state of deep sedation, I sprayed his throat and nose with a local anesthetic to diminish any discomfort as I passed a thin, black, flexible fiberoptic tube through his nose to visualize his airways. As the scope was advanced, the vocal cords came into view. I watched as his cords slowly separated and closed in sync with each inspiration and expiration. Passing the scope through the vocal cords was often met with vigorous coughing and sudden shortness of breath. On occasion, the vocal cords would go into spasm and close off the airway. To diminish the likelihood of vocal cord spasm, I squirted additional local anesthetic through the scope directly onto the cords. After a few seconds, I gently passed the thin fiberoptic scope between the vocal cords and entered the windpipe, known as the trachea. I paused for a few seconds to make sure that Jonathan remained comfortable. After a few coughs, and another dose of Versed, the procedure continued.

Jonathan's breathing remained steady and unlabored. His oxygen monitor and heart monitor showed stable vital signs. The anesthesiologist made sure that additional sedation was provided as needed. I then focused on the task at hand of visualizing the inside of Jonathan's bronchial tubes. I was looking for any abnormalities such as tumors, plugs of mucus, or purple spots of Kaposi's sarcoma, another AIDS-defining illness. I was rather convinced that Jonathan had AIDS. I gently passed the bronchoscope and made twists and turns in the various segmental airways by rotating my wrist and pressing a lever upward or downward with my thumb. With simultaneous twisting of the wrist and movement of the thumb, I could guide the scope down the various branching paths of the tracheobronchial tree.

Visualization only took a few minutes. The airways were without obstruction and no signs of Kaposi's sarcoma were evident. The secretions were thin and watery. To this day, I remain amazed that virtually all tracheobronchial trees share the same anatomical features with rare exceptions. Although there are two lungs, the right and left lungs are not identical. The right lung contains the right upper lobe, right middle lobe, and right lower lobe. The left lung contains the left upper lobe and the left lower lobe. Although one might think otherwise, the right lung airways and the left lung airways are not symmetrical.

After thorough inspection of Jonathan's airways, I wedged the scope in a bronchial tube of the left upper lobe and my assistant instilled 50 cc of sterile saline through a side port on the fiberoptic device. Through the lens of the scope, I could see the saline entering the airways. Seconds later, I squeezed my thumb on the suction channel and watched as cloudy fluid emanated from the airways and filled a small plastic container attached to the scope. After collecting samples, I gradually removed the scope and the procedure was completed. Jonathan was wheeled to the recovery room for post-procedure monitoring.

Even to this day, having performed over 1,000 fiberoptic bronchoscopic procedures, a sense of extreme hypervigilance is with me from start to finish. Although confident in my skills, I never lose sight of the fact that the life of another human being is in my hands during this procedure. Although death during bronchoscopy is rare, it can occur, related to the anesthetic, bleeding, or a collapsed lung.

Jonathan's procedure went very smoothly. As always, I personally hand-delivered the bronchoscopic specimens to the lab. I would not allow for the possibility that one of these specimens could be lost in transit. Soon thereafter, I received a call from the lab that indeed the specimen showed the classic appearance of squished Ping-Pong balls, pathognomonic for pneumocystis. Jonathan was diagnosed with pneumocystis carinii pneumonia and, accordingly, AIDS.

In our Center City hospital, pneumocystis carinii pneumonia was diagnosed almost daily in the mid to late 1980s. We were at the epicenter of the AIDS epidemic, and

I was often called upon to perform bronchoscopy to confirm the diagnosis and guide treatment. Our staff had become very skilled in diagnosing and managing AIDS and its associated opportunistic infections.

As I headed for the elevator to start daily rounds, my beeper sounded. I was paged STAT to the recovery room. Jonathan was in respiratory distress. The cardiac monitor revealed extreme tachycardia, an increase in his heart rate. His oxygen saturation was dropping. The progressive change in tone of the pulse oximeter alarm signaled grave danger. I knew something was seriously wrong. The procedure had gone so well and yet Jonathan could die within minutes without a correct diagnosis and intervention.

A STAT chest X-ray obtained failed to show evidence of lung collapse. Then the vital clue surfaced. Blood was drawn from the radial artery of Jonathan's wrist to determine blood pH, and carbon dioxide and oxygen levels. The color was neither bright red as seen in a patient with a normal oxygen level, nor was it dark red as seen in a patient with a low oxygen level.

Instead, the blood was brown! The patient was cyanotic, that is, with bluish discoloration. With the brown-colored blood and the patient colored blue, this could only be seen in the rare condition known as methemoglobinemia. Jonathan's hemoglobin molecules that carry oxygen throughout his body had been altered by a reaction to the local anesthetic used to numb his airways. Systemic absorption of this medication is usually minimal. However, enough medication had been absorbed to change the iron element that binds oxygen in the hemoglobin molecule. Because of the change in the iron molecule, it could no longer bind oxygen.

If Jonathan's condition were not immediately reversed, he would soon die. A blood test confirmed the diagnosis. Sixty percent of his hemoglobin molecules had been transformed into a physiologic state incapable of binding oxygen. That left only 40 percent of his hemoglobin to deliver oxygen to all the cells of his vital organs. The antidote, methylene blue, was infused through Jonathan's intravenous line. Iron molecules in his hemoglobin were converted back to a normal state capable of binding oxygen. Jonathan's bluish discoloration resolved quickly.

Blue Patient, Brown Blood

As is often the case, Jonathan did not recall what had transpired. The amnesiac quality of the sedative rendered him incapable of remembering the procedure and scary life-threatening events that followed. Within hours, Jonathan was fully awake and breathing comfortably.

I returned to Jonathan's room that evening and informed him of the day's events and that he had been diagnosed with an AIDS-defining illness known as pneumocystis carinii pneumonia. He began to cry as he acknowledged that he had suspected this was the case. Reality was setting in.

Jonathan responded very well to his twenty-one-day course of the antibiotic Bactrim, as well as the steroid prednisone, to treat the inflammation in his lungs. On the day of his hospital discharge, he noted marked improvement in his breathing. He no longer needed oxygen supplementation, and his shortness of breath had completely resolved. He was delighted to breathe normally again but clearly apprehensive about his new diagnosis of AIDS.

An infectious disease consultant spoke with Jonathan on the day of discharge, arranged for outpatient follow-up, and initiation of antiretroviral therapy. I never saw Jonathan again but remain hopeful to this day that he fulfilled his dream of becoming a great conductor. I, too, hoped that he would continue to benefit from the miraculous medical breakthroughs brought about by great cooperation among industry, government, and scientists to ultimately turn AIDS from a certain premature death into a chronic condition with an excellent prognosis.

25

Heart Attack

For years, James was informed by his doctors that without a change in behaviors, he was headed for trouble. Although he had no control over his strong family history of premature coronary artery disease, he certainly could alter his eating habits and sedentary lifestyle.

James was home, watching TV. It was the 9th inning and the Phillies were losing by three runs. James was getting drowsy and considering going to bed. Suddenly, the bases were loaded, and James's drowsiness turned to excitement. With three balls and two strikes, all the fans in the stadium (and James at home) were on their feet. Then, in a moment of drama a baseball game can provide, the batter swung at a low-hanging curve ball and drove it over the left field wall for a walk-off grand-slam home run. The Phillies had come from behind to win the game.

Suddenly, James began to feel short of breath. A frightening sensation overwhelmed him as he began to sweat profusely. He fell back into the recliner but maintained consciousness. His wife was sleeping soundly on the second floor. James knew immediately that he was having a heart attack. He began to cry as thoughts of death overwhelmed him.

He screamed for Helen, his wife of thirty-nine years. James and Helen grew up in the same South Philadelphia neighborhood. They were high school sweethearts and practically inseparable except for when the Phillies were on television. For years, Helen had tried to convince James to stop eating cheesesteaks and exercise more regularly. James had been very athletic and trim as a youth, but sports-related knee injuries led to increasing time spent watching television and gradual weight gain. Although weighing just 160 pounds in high school, he now tipped the scales at 295. Helen panicked at the first sight of her adoring husband. She knew that something was very wrong.

Paramedics arrived within minutes. Blood pressure and heart rate were elevated, and oxygen saturation level was decreased. James denied chest pain but did inform the paramedics that he felt short of breath. He was placed on a stretcher and carefully taken to the ambulance. Helen squeezed his hand and would not let go. She held back her tears and prayed that she would not lose the love of her life. The events to follow would be in the hands of total strangers. Helen could only pray that the paramedics would drive safely and quickly to the right hospital, a hospital fully equipped to treat a heart attack with up-to-date interventions in a timely manner.

Henry, the lead paramedic, reassured James and Helen that James would get great care at Pennsylvania Hospital, the nation's first. This modern-day center, founded by Benjamin Franklin at a time when bloodletting was in vogue, was well equipped to care for James in this moment of great need. After Henry placed an intravenous line in James and gave him nasal oxygen prongs, Henry reviewed the EKG obtained by his partner, Alice.

James was having a STEMI, (ST-Elevation Myocardial Infarction), a heart attack, caused by the complete obstruction of one of his major coronary arteries. The clock was ticking. With every minute's delay in opening the vessel came a greater risk of permanent heart impairment or death.

Alice called the Pennsylvania Hospital emergency department and informed them, "We have a fifty-nine-year-old obese male with stable vital signs having a STEMI." This pronouncement activated a highly regulated chain of events. The cardiac catheterization team, with its lead invasive cardiology specialist, nurses, and technicians, would need to drop everything and go immediately to the cardiac cath lab in preparation for James's arrival.

After Alice hung up the phone, she wiped James's sweaty brow and gave him four chewable baby aspirins. Ironically, this pill, named for the youngsters it was meant to treat, is more commonly consumed by adults for stroke and heart attacks. Its potent anti-platelet activity helps prevent aggregation of small blood cells known to adhere to the insides of coronary vessels and block the flow of blood. Although usually given prophylactically to prevent a second stroke or heart attack, its use in an emergency such as this has become the standard of care. Within minutes, James was wheeled into the emergency room with Helen's hand firmly attached to his.

Dr. Wilson had trained many years for moments like this. She knew during high school that she would follow in the footsteps of her mother and become a cardiologist. Although her mother was a noninvasive cardiologist, Dr. Wilson enjoyed the excitement of cardiac catheterization. She had signed up for a life filled with disruptions: interrupted sporting events and piano recitals. She sometimes wondered if the thrill would fade with time or if the burdens of a disrupted life would eventually overwhelm her.

Little did James and Helen appreciate in the moment that healthcare providers from around the city had been alerted and were about to descend on James's bedside in the cardiac cath lab. In the emergency room, James was given several standard cardiac medications and quickly wheeled down the hall to be prepped for the procedure that would determine his fate.

The goal was ninety minutes to revascularization. A delay in opening James's clogged coronary artery would diminish his chance of survival. James and Helen were fortunate that they lived in a city with multiple major health centers only minutes away. Helen was trying to stay positive and jokingly told James it was a good thing they had not retired to a small town in Florida.

Peggy, the cardiac nurse, turned to Helen: "Time to say good-bye." As Helen let go of James's hand, she could not stop the floodgate of tears from opening. She bent over to kiss his forehead, wondering if it would be the last time.

Helen clearly grasped the gravity of the situation. She had watched her father die of a sudden massive heart attack when she was a young teen. That vision often haunted her, and she frequently wondered whether her father would still be alive if he had had access to today's miraculous medical interventions. While Helen sat in the waiting area, she called each of their three adult children. As none had ever left South Philly, they all arrived at the hospital within the hour. James and Helen had raised three children with love and devotion. They had remained a very close family and went to church together every Sunday.

Dr. Wilson introduced herself to James as she began to prep for the procedure. A technician shaved James's groin and applied a Betadine solution to prevent infection. Within minutes, James was in a twilight state induced by a mild sedative administered by anesthesia. Dr. Wilson threaded a catheter through the femoral artery and advanced it under fluoroscopy, a form of continuous X-ray. She injected a material known as contrast so the blocked artery could be visualized prior to placing a stent. Determining the exact site of the blockage was essential.

Suddenly, Peggy alerted Dr. Wilson that James was in V-tach, a heart rhythm disorder or arrhythmia know as ventricular tachycardia. Normally, rhythmic signals of electrical activity begin in the sinus node of the right atrium. Then the signals spread to other regions of the heart so that the ventricles, the two largest heart chambers, contract in a coordinated manner to effectively expel oxygen-rich blood to all the cells of the body. Here, James's normal sinus rhythm had been replaced by this rapid dysfunctional rhythm originating in an irritated oxygen-deprived cell of one of the ventricles.

This was a direct consequence of the heart attack James was experiencing. He was at risk for cardiac arrest leading to sudden death. Without skipping a beat, Dr. Wilson yelled, "Clear," as she applied an electrical shock to the heart with a defibrillator. As quickly as James had gone into V-tach, he resumed normal sinus rhythm and stabilization of his vital signs. Dr. Wilson placed a stent in the left anterior descending artery, known as the widowmaker vessel.

As James was wheeled to recovery, Dr. Wilson headed to the waiting room. Helen and the children knew that things had gone well when Dr Wilson walked through the door with a great smile and two thumbs up.

Later that night, while James was still in the recovery room with Helen and their kids, he asked what Dr. Wilson had told them. None of them remembered the exact words but only the joy they immediately felt on learning that their loved one was going to be okay. James pledged to change his lifestyle. Helen said, "You better or I will kill you!" They all laughed until they cried.

Over the past fifty years, we have witnessed dramatic advances in our lifesaving capabilities. With the invention of the defibrillator and pacemaker, pioneered by Boston cardiologist Dr. Paul Zoll, widespread construction of coronary care units and centralized care of critically ill patients followed.

These dedicated units allow for continuous cardiac monitoring of patients most vulnerable for cardiac arrest. Physicians and nurses who specialize in cardiac care respond within seconds to hearts that stop beating. Application of electrical shock, medications, and, if necessary, cardiac compression can resuscitate a heart that would otherwise cease to function forever.

In parallel with dissemination of coronary care units came the evolution of medical and surgical intensive care units for the management of noncardiac medical and surgical critically ill patients. These patients are evaluated frequently for alterations in vital signs by highly dedicated and well-trained healthcare providers.

According to the CDC, heart disease is the leading cause of death in the United States and coronary artery disease is the most common disorder of the heart. Eighteen million adults suffer from significant atherosclerotic narrowing of the coronary arteries. Almost one million Americans each year suffer a heart attack, also known as a myocardial infarction. Risk factors include:

- Cigarette smoking
- Obesity
- Diabetes mellitus
- Hyperlipidemia (elevated cholesterol)

- Hypertension
- Inactivity
- Positive family history
- Undiagnosed/untreated obstructive sleep apnea

Patients with atherosclerosis of the coronary arteries are at risk for developing a life-threatening heart attack when a plaque ruptures in one of the teeny heart-nourishing coronary vessels. Such a sudden rupture may occur spontaneously or following extreme emotion, strenuous exercise, exposure to a cold environment, or sexual activity. The prototypic disastrous exercise is the shoveling of snow during freezing temperatures. The combination of exercise and a cold environment may be deadly.

Rupture of a plaque within a coronary artery exposes components of the vessel wall lining and activates the formation of a blood clot. With sudden subsequent coronary obstruction, a decrease in oxygen delivery to heart muscle cells served by the vessel, tissue necrosis/cell death follows, and leakage of cardiac enzymes into the blood signifies the development of a heart attack. For some, the oxygen-deprived heart cells become arrhythmogenic—tending to lead to an arrhythmia—and ventricular tachycardia or ventricular fibrillation may follow. This may result in sudden cardiac death.

For those fortunate enough to survive this potentially deadly event and arrive alive in the emergency room with an EKG showing ST-segment elevations, a STEMI is diagnosed. Revascularization (opening the occluded coronary vessel) with a percutaneous coronary intervention (stent placement) within ninety minutes leads to a dramatically increased probability of survival with preservation of heart muscle function and to an ultimate resumption of a normal life.

Subsequent long-term follow-up with a cardiologist is essential for medical management to diminish the risk of a second, potentially fatal, heart attack. Medical management will certainly include lifelong aspirin therapy as an anti-platelet agent as well as statin therapy for aggressive control of lipids circulating in the bloodstream and other cardiac medications as determined by the cardiologist.

26

Wheezes

Rebecca had outgrown her childhood asthma and never gave it a second thought until she moved to Philadelphia. After a period of asymptomatic years, her wheezing returned. She suspected her dusty, moldy apartment was a significant contributing factor.

Asthma has a worldwide prevalence of approximately 7–10 percent. Despite major advances in treatment, thousands die every year in the United States from this disease of the airways characterized by inflammation and dysfunction of airway smooth muscles. Contributing factors to death from asthma include failure to recognize severity of the disease, failure to treat the inflammation of the airways, poor access to healthcare, and environmental exposures that trigger airflow obstruction.

An individual with poorly controlled asthma generally experiences breathlessness, wheezing, and chest tightness. Although short-acting bronchodilators such as albuterol are effective in relieving acute symptoms, they do not address the underlying inflammatory process that contributes chronically to the airway narrowing. Without a doubt, corticosteroids have been lifesaving in the management of asthma. A five-day course of an oral steroid such as prednisone can rapidly transform a patient suffering from extreme breathlessness due to airflow obstruction to one who is functioning normally.

However, chronic use of systemic steroids contributes to adverse side effects such as osteoporosis, avascular necrosis of the bone, cataracts, diabetes, and increased vulnerability to infection. Undoubtedly, the greatest advance in the management of asthma has been the development of the inhaled corticosteroid. By inhaling the steroid, it allows for maximum effect in the targeted airways with a decrease in systemic absorption and, therefore, fewer systemic side effects.

An inhaled corticosteroid, alone or in combination with a long-acting bronchodilator known as a beta agonist, often serves as maintenance treatment and allows most patients to live normal functioning lives. Today, this brilliant combination drug has revolutionized the management of asthma. Its development by the pharmaceutical industry followed research demonstrating that underlying inflammation leads to swelling of the bronchial tubes. This in conjunction with dysfunction of the surrounding smooth muscles, contributes to airway narrowing. This results in airway bronchoconstriction culminating in the universal asthmatic symptoms of cough, wheezing, and shortness of breath.

In the subset of patients with significant allergies, consultation with an allergist may prove beneficial. Avoidance of identified allergens and desensitization with allergy shots may be of value. A pill known as a leukotriene modifier may be added to an inhaled corticosteroid/long-acting beta agonist regimen if asthma symptoms are not adequately controlled.

Patients with Samter's Triad—asthma, aspirin sensitivity, and nasal polyps—a type of AERD (Aspirin Exacerbated Respiratory Disease), may show clinical improvement with a leukotriene modifier. Treatment of coexistent reflux and sinus disease as well as attention to contributing environmental factors also prove beneficial.

Patients with chronic asthma often benefit from an individually tailored asthma action plan. The patient uses a plastic device known as a peak flow meter to monitor airflow and is provided with a plan to intervene with a step-up in therapy based upon written instructions provided by a clinician. Some patients benefit from new biologics such as anti-IgE and anti-interleukin-5 injections if the serum IgE or absolute eosinophil count is elevated. Despite proper treatment, some patients will deteriorate to the point of requiring hospitalization where more aggressive inhalational and systemic steroid treatment may be administered. It is the rare patient who requires a brief course of mechanical ventilation for severe refractory life-threatening asthma.

When I first met Rebecca, her asthma was easily controlled with a combination inhaler containing an inhaled corticosteroid and a long-acting beta agonist (a bronchodilator that opens the airway.) In addition, Rebecca always carried an albuterol inhaler in her purse. She knew to use it for rescue. She had an action plan that allowed her to self-medicate in response to drops in her peak flow measured by a small inexpensive plastic device she would blow into each day to assess airway function.

Rebecca called me on a Monday morning. She had been experiencing wheezes and shortness of breath all weekend and had been using her nebulizer with increased frequency. Based on her asthma action plan, and in accordance with her drop in peak flow, she had initiated therapy with prednisone, a potent systemic steroid. Rebecca expressed embarrassment that with the loss of her job, she could no longer afford her costly but lifesaving inhaled corticosteroid/long-acting beta agonist she had used as her daily maintenance inhaler and had been without the device for two weeks but delayed calling me because of her embarrassment.

Because Rebecca could not complete sentences without gasping or sucking in air, it was obvious that immediate hospitalization was necessary. I met Rebecca in our hospital's emergency department within the hour. Her peak flow upon arrival was 25 percent of her baseline. This signified severe airway narrowing due to poorly controlled asthma and progressive airway inflammation. Undoubtedly, Rebecca's inability to afford her inhaler was the primary cause of this life-threatening event.

Wheezes

Rebecca was breathing albuterol, a short-acting bronchodilator, continuously through a nebulizer upon my arrival. She had been given a large dose of an intravenous steroid with the hope that treatment would kick in before her respiratory muscles fatigued. Knowing that asthmatics have a decreased chance of survival if placed on a ventilator, we were very hopeful that these interventions would suffice. However, Rebecca was showing signs that intubation might be required for ventilatory support in the next few hours if she did not show significant improvement.

As a last-ditch effort, the mixture of inhaled gas she was breathing through a mask providing 50 percent oxygen/50 percent nitrogen was changed to 50 percent oxygen/50 percent helium. We normally breathe air that has 20.9 percent oxygen and approximately 79 percent nitrogen. The nitrogen is inert and just goes along for the ride without any clinical benefit or harm. By replacing nitrogen with helium, a gas with less density, the work of breathing in an acute asthmatic exacerbation is often diminished.

Rebecca made it through the night with continuous albuterol and the oxygen/helium gas mixture while she was closely monitored by nurses in the intensive care unit. However, the following morning, her condition worsened. Her breathing became more labored and her respiratory rate more rapid. She was extremely breathless and moving little air with each breath. She had visible retractions of her neck as she used accessory muscles to supplement her fatiguing diaphragm. After discussion with Rebecca, we decided to proceed with placement of an endotracheal tube in her trachea for attachment to a mechanical ventilator.

Once on the ventilator, we heavily sedated Rebecca and initiated therapy with a muscle paralytic for better control of her dysfunctional breathing pattern. Her brain was continuing to send electrical messages to her diaphragm at a rapid rate in response to the airway narrowing. However, her airways needed more time to exhale each breath through tightly narrowed, diffusely inflamed bronchial tubes. With the use of a paralytic, we were able to control her respiratory rate and allow more time for exhalation to prevent stacking of breaths, which happens if a subsequent breath is initiated prior to complete exhalation of the previous one. This stacking can result in an increase in intrathoracic pressure acting like a vise squeezing around the chest which could then cause a decrease in blood return to the heart, and a drop in blood pressure with ultimate cardiovascular collapse. This process, known as dynamic hyperinflation, can lead to death.

As each day passed, Rebecca's condition improved, and the paralytic was stopped. Her sedation was lightened. Her critical care nurses remained hypervigilant around the clock and provided her medications as well as basic needs, including personal hygiene and frequent turning. A respiratory therapist checked the digital readout of her ventilator to ensure proper functioning, and to troubleshoot as alarms sounded frequently. During the COVID-19 pandemic, these are the same therapists who risked their lives through potential exposure to large viral loads capable of causing death.

On the day of her liberation from mechanical ventilation, Rebecca expressed gratitude toward everyone who had helped her through this traumatic episode. Indeed, it was an event that could potentially lead to post-traumatic stress disorder characterized by nightmares and flashbacks.

Something as simple as an inhaler, unaffordable to Rebecca, would have prevented this life-threatening medical crisis and certainly would have been significantly less costly to our healthcare system. A classic example of penny wise and dollar foolish. I left the hospital that day wondering how many would have to die before we legislate affordable healthcare for all. We need not reinvent the wheel. We should simply look to the north at our Canadian neighbors or across the Atlantic to our European allies to find a solution to this healthcare crisis. We need to address the issue of why we as a nation spend more per capita on healthcare than most and yet get significantly less in return. Affordable healthcare for all is a basic human right.

27

Anaphylaxis

Jill was so excited that she was finally going to watch the Eagles football game in person. It was Sunday morning and she and her husband were preparing food for the pregame tailgate "ceremony." Friends with season tickets were unable to attend, so Jill and her husband were the lucky recipients of these highly valued seats. She dressed head to toe in Eagle colors and even adorned her face with green makeup. Although she had grown up in a football family who watched the NFL every Sunday, she had never actually been to a game. She recalled with great affection Sundays with her father and brothers during her childhood.

As she was locking the front door, Jill popped her antibiotic pill for her strep throat as she had done previously without any side effects. This easily treatable infection was once the cause of deadly kidney failure, and rheumatic fever leading to progressive valvular destruction and heart failure. I often reflect upon the great loss of life prior to the discovery of penicillin and other antimicrobials and express gratitude for these amazing advances in medicine that have saved so many lives.

While driving on the Schuylkill Expressway, Jill began to experience a diffuse itch from head to toe. Her husband, Tom, noticed hives that had distorted Jill's facial features. She exclaimed that she was fine though she knew she was not. Tom turned onto 8th Street and declared, "We are going to Pennsylvania Hospital." Though initially reluctant and somewhat argumentative, Jill acquiesced and responded, "We can still make it to the game by kickoff."

Upon arrival to the emergency department, Jill's hives and facial swelling had progressed. Her lips and tongue had become swollen. The triage nurse quickly placed Jill in a cubicle for urgent physician evaluation. Within minutes, Dr. Cressman introduced himself. By now, Jill could not speak. The swelling of her lips and tongue had progressed to involve the back of her throat. As she sucked in air, a loud stridorous wheeze was audible across the room with each inspiration.

Jill's blood pressure was markedly reduced at 60/40 and her heart rate was high at 140. It was quickly evident, without further history or testing, that Jill was experiencing anaphylactic shock due to a life-threatening allergic reaction to her antibiotic. Without immediate treatment, this young Eagles fan would be dead.

Would the medical team make a quick diagnosis and intervene with the correct treatment? There was no time for additional questions, examination, or testing. In quick succession, Dr. Cressman gave Nurse Andrews orders for intramuscular epinephrine; one liter of lactated Ringer's intravenous fluid; 125 mg IV Solu-medrol, a potent steroid; and 50 mg of IV Benadryl, an antihistamine.

Within three minutes, Jill's facial, lip, tongue, and throat swelling began to resolve. Her voice returned to normal, and her breathing became unlabored. Within ten minutes, her blood pressure and heart rate were back to normal. Jill looked at her watch: it was 12:30 P.M. She turned to Tom and proclaimed, "We still have time to make it before kickoff." Dr. Cressman and Nurse Andrews looked at each other and briefly nodded and chuckled. "You will be watching the game from your ICU bed."

Jill could not understand why she should be hospitalized, much less in the ICU. She now felt fine. Dr. Cressman, now with a calm demeanor and soft-spoken voice, explained that Jill had experienced life-threatening anaphylactic shock from antibiotic ingestion. Jill's highly evolved immune system, normally protecting her from hostile microbes, had mistakenly identified this lifesaving antibiotic as a foreign invader. This led to the release of immunoglobulin troops that attached to spherical balls known as mast cells. Subsequent release of vasoactive substances such as histamine caused the airway swelling that nearly led to death by asphyxiation.

Dr. Cressman further explained that approximately one-third of patients experience a life-threatening relapse within twenty-four hours of initial treatment. There was no choice but to admit Jill to the ICU for further monitoring. She was deeply saddened by the missed opportunity but expressed gratitude that her life-threatening allergic reaction had resolved as she was transported by wheelchair to the intensive care unit, still in her green Eagles attire. Tom held her hand as he contemplated the near loss of his life partner and the quick interventions that had saved her.

28

Blackout

My wife and I had looked forward to dining out with our son for weeks. He was a medical intern and his eighty-hour work week limited our opportunities to spend time together. On this night, while dining at one of our favorite local Italian restaurants, our son was recapping some of his recent training experiences. Just after ordering our entrees, I witnessed out of the corner of my eye one of the waiters drop to the floor.

My son saw it also. Without hesitation, he and I jumped from our seats and ran to assist the fallen man. As we kneeled beside the waiter, I watched with great pride as my son began to question him about his medical history. A gash above his right eyebrow required pressure with what had been a clean white table linen. It became clear that the waiter had been experiencing recurrent bouts of syncope, the medical term for blacking out. This time, he struck his head on a vertical wrought iron pole that decorated this lovely dining room. We assessed his ABCs: airway, breathing, and circulation. He was clearly breathing and had a strong regular pulse. As my son turned to another waiter and instructed him to call 911, the patient lying on the floor, appearing cold and clammy, yelled "No!" He adamantly refused to go to the emergency room.

We later speculated that he had no insurance and could not afford the costly bills that would follow an emergency room visit and hospitalization. As a competent adult, he had the right to refuse treatment, but he promised to call his primary care physician for further follow-up. After two blood-soaked linens were applied firmly to his wound, he stopped bleeding. He slowly stood up and went back to work in the restaurant kitchen.

As my son and I slowly ventured back to our table, an intense feeling of disappointment, brought on by a missed opportunity to secure hospital care for this fallen gentleman, was replaced by a feeling of joy. Almost forty years after I had provided a lifesaving thump, which I described in chapter one, to a patient with syncope, my kind, gentle son, now a physician, was prepared to carry the baton. He and many youthful, newly minted physicians I have had the great privilege of training would now use their skills and compassion to attend to the sick and injured and relieve their breathlessness.

29

Self-Compassion
by Batsirai Bvunzawabaya, Ph.D.

My first meeting with Dr. Kotler was on a tennis court, not as his patient. That came later. I was nervous about playing doubles with a group of people I had never met. I was assured that it would be fun, but I was skeptical. As a person skilled at hiding my shyness, and presenting in a (hopefully) warm demeanor, I often enter new spaces with a cautious optimism. At that time, it was hard to know that not only would Dr. Kotler diagnose and treat my asthma, but it was the beginning of a great relationship between healthcare professionals.

Becoming a counseling psychologist is probably one of the most meaningful life decisions that I have ever made. Building a strong relationship with my patients, I experience some of the joys of seeing them abandon unhelpful and sometimes harmful life patterns and discover inner strengths that lay dormant. We see new relationships taking shape and movement toward major life decisions. As a psychotherapist, building a strong relationship can be life changing for both parties, as it facilitates growth, empathy, and compassion.

Compassion is a deep concern that moves us toward a desire to alleviate another's suffering. It is the driving force behind the work of any great caregiver. For social workers, psychologists, nurses, physicians, home health aides, and various other healthcare providers, our work can feel like a calling, a part of our identity. It is humbling to be part of another's existence as they make difficult life decisions, receive urgent medical care, and, at times, while they mourn their losses.

Kristin Neff, Ph.D. is widely recognized as one of the world's leading experts on self-compassion. She has written extensively on the topic, the act of applying a compassionate stance toward ourselves. She highlights the need for kindness and warmth toward our own struggles, recognizing that we suffer in the same way as others, and she encourages people to observe their emotions in a balanced manner, also known as mindfulness. Self-compassion requires that we resist criticizing or judging ourselves, exaggerating or minimizing our emotions, or seeing our pain as something we alone experience. This may sound simple, but it is incredibly difficult to refrain from "evaluating" ourselves during a time of great stress.

Part of being autonomous is knowing when to ask for help.

John R. Atherton, MS, LMHP, MAC
Psychotherapist

The relationship between a healthcare provider and the patient is made up of brief yet meaningful interactions. Rapport must develop expeditiously, at a time when patients and their loved ones are at their most vulnerable. Trust can occur instantly in emergency situations, as the patient hopes their suffering will be taken seriously and that they can be cured. As healthcare providers, when our patients suffer, on some level we do, too. We may not focus on our suffering while we are performing our duties, but it is always present in the back of our minds. It is natural to postpone expressing and coping with our own suffering because the needs of our patients are immediate.

During the COVID-19 pandemic of 2020, healthcare providers across a wide spectrum have experienced this intensity of need in very significant ways. They risked their lives, postponed the expression of their own emotions and at times their grief. They went without much-needed rest and self-care in order to meet the high demands of their professions. The physical and emotional isolation required in the treatment of COVID-19 separated patients from their loved ones and affirmed the sacred role of healthcare providers. In a lot of cases, the last person the patient saw or heard was their healthcare provider.

Existential anxiety is embedded in the healthcare provider role. Am I enough? Will the support and knowledge I possess be sufficient for patients and their loved ones? We demand so much from ourselves, and we must. The painful reality is, even when we perform above and beyond the standard of care, lives can be lost. There is no training that makes this easier. Whether the loss is due to a long-standing illness, an accident, or suicide, the psychological impact on the loved ones and healthcare providers can be devastating. After losing a patient or a loved one, a deep sense of loss occurs. At such times, it is important to be self-compassionate and to extend the care we normally give to others to ourselves.

Sometimes the role of caregiver can extend into a healthcare provider's personal life. For instance, family members may describe their ailments in hopes of a quick diagnosis and treatment recommendations. Or, while engaged in treatment, loved ones may check in to see whether the medical guidance they have received is accurate. Because it is hard to resist the urge to share knowledge that can be helpful to those around us, the lack of a complete break between work and life demands can lead healthcare providers to feel that they are always on the clock. Without adequate boundaries one's internal resources can become depleted, and neglect of our own physical, emotional, social, and psychological needs can occur where our ability to continue to give great care to others is compromised. I have fallen into this pattern myself, believing that if I just work a little harder, give a little more support to others, I can rest later.

When helpers overidentify with the emotions or physical suffering of others, compassion fatigue (an experience of traumatic stress in the helper) can arise. Burnout is a prolonged work-related stress that results in a feeling of emptiness, and mental, physical, and emotional exhaustion. It also results in reduced job satisfaction, which can create a deficiency in meeting the daily demands of life.

While providing patient care in high-stress situations, healthcare professionals also cope with their own personal life challenges: professional accountability measures, inadequate institutional support, and sleep deprivation, along with other stressors. A healthcare provider can find themselves feeling intense sadness and anxiety, hopelessness, social withdrawal, mood fluctuations, helplessness, difficulty with concentration and memory, indecisiveness, and thoughts of death. Physically, they may experience low energy, body aches, increased heart rate, sweating, restlessness, and trouble breathing. Many of these can be signs of depression or anxiety but can also signal the presence of other mental health diagnoses.

Those caring for loved ones are not immune to the mental health concerns experienced by healthcare providers. In fact, any individual who has faced previous traumatic experiences, and those predisposed to mental health challenges, may be vulnerable to encountering these mental illnesses. For people with a family member or a friend who is chronically ill, or is having a medical emergency, compassion is usually present in abundance. In those moments, loved ones are often shouldering the worries of the patient while holding on to hope, reciting prayers of healing and encouraging those around them to do the same. This is typically a time of uncertainty, anxiety, and grief. For family members there can be feelings of guilt and shame about feeling burdened by the responsibility of caring for a loved one. It can be difficult to recognize those emotions and address them during a loved one's illness because we are preoccupied with "being there" for our loved one.

Family members caring for critically ill loved ones may feel internal pressure to quiet feelings of anger, shame, or fear with expressions of gratitude for the parts of their lives that are untouched by hardship. Identifying difficult emotions can feel like a "betrayal" to their loved ones or to a higher power even though these reactions are understandable when caring for someone who is critically ill. Sometimes, there is a worry that if they open the door to some of these difficult and painful emotions, their reactions will be destructive and hard to contain. The idea of being compassionate toward one's self in those moments can be perceived as self-indulgent. Expressing that we feel tired, frustrated, or hopeless can bring about feelings of guilt, particularly when our suffering coincides with times when others close to us are hurting. As a result, it can be challenging to have family members find comfort in expressing these feelings while still maintaining compassion for themselves.

We often internalize negative attitudes and carry shame about seeking help for mental health concerns. There can sometimes be public stigma or negative attitudes in society directed at those who experience trouble with their mental health. Aspects of our sociocultural identities such as gender, racial and ethnic background, sexual orientation, religious affiliation, and social class can influence our views on mental health and whether we seek help. It is a common misconception that not needing support for mental health is a sign of strength.

Even though this is inaccurate, we can be inclined to cope with difficulties in isolation. Issues with mental health are typically a normal reaction to life stressors, and we have a long way to go in recognizing, accepting, and normalizing this reality. For healthcare providers, concerns about judgment, limited time for self-care, and confidentiality concerns may be added barriers to seeking support. For marginalized communities, such as people of color, trusting and finding providers who share in their identities and experiences, and for low-income communities, access to care may present additional challenges. Stigma not only directly affects individuals with mental health concerns but also the loved ones who support them due to worries about disclosing the mental health needs within their families.

Addressing the challenges of caring for others while maintaining self-compassion can be complicated. It requires self-awareness and practice. Engaging in psychotherapy, religious or spiritual groups, or any communities that affirms its members in a meaningful way are avenues to gaining self-compassion skills. We are, after all, social animals. Allowing ourselves and those around us permission to discuss how we feel provides helpful modeling and normalizes the wide range of reactions that can arise as a caregiver or family member. During times of providing care to others, self-care practices such as mindfulness, journaling, or spending time in nature can also provide avenues to emotional healing.

In Closing

Now in the twilight of my career, I find myself reflecting on the great courage I have witnessed in patients and their families as they endured the suffering of critical illness. I contemplate the generosity of countless providers with whom I have had the privilege and pleasure of working, and who, without agenda other than to heal and support, delivered healthcare with empathy and compassion. I am struck by the tremendous advances brought about by innovative technologies leading to lifesaving interventions and prolonged longevity when applied with wisdom and in accordance with patients' goals and priorities.

These observations reaffirm for me a life well lived as a medical doctor caring for those afflicted with severe disease. Although not without great challenges, physically and emotionally, this journey of learning, teaching, and caring has been well worth the many sacrifices along the way. In the end, life is all about forming loving relationships anchored by empathy and compassion. These are the lessons I have learned over many years as husband, father, grandfather, son, brother, uncle, colleague, friend, teacher, and physician.

About the Author

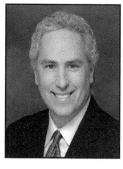

Ronald Kotler, M.D., is a pulmonologist who specializes in breathing disorders. He received his bachelor's degree in chemistry at Emory University in Atlanta, Georgia, where he was elected to the Phi Beta Kappa academic honor society. He obtained his medical degree at the University of Pennsylvania School of Medicine in Philadelphia, Pennsylvania, where he was elected to the Alpha Omega Alpha Honor Medical Society. After training in internal medicine at Pennsylvania Hospital, he completed a fellowship in pulmonary diseases at the Hospital of the University of Pennsylvania in Philadelphia.

After completing his fellowship, he spent decades as a pulmonary/critical care medicine specialist. Dr. Kotler cofounded the Pennsylvania Hospital Sleep Disorders Center, where he is currently the medical director. His primary interest is in the evaluation and treatment of patients with sleep-related breathing disorders. He has been elected to fellowships in the American College of Physicians, American College of Chest Physicians, and the American Academy of Sleep Medicine.

Dr. Kotler is a clinical professor of medicine at the University of Pennsylvania and enjoys teaching pulmonary pathophysiology to second-year medical students. He is the coauthor of *365 Ways to Get a Good Night's Sleep* and contributor to the *New York Times* best seller, *20 Years Younger.* He has appeared on *Good Morning America* and *The Oprah Winfrey Show.*

Dr. Kotler lives in Philadelphia with his wife, Jane, and enjoys spending quality time with his three children, their spouses, and eight grandchildren. He is an avid tennis player and enjoys all sports.